Health as Expanding Consciousness

Second Edition

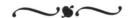

NLN
PRESS

Health as Expanding Consciousness

Second Edition

Margaret A. Newman
PhD, RN, FAAN

Professor, School of Nursing
University of Minnesota
Minneapolis, Minnesota

JONES AND BARTLETT PUBLISHERS
Sudbury, Massachusetts
BOSTON   TORONTO   LONDON   SINGAPORE

World Headquarters
Jones and Bartlett Publishers
40 Tall Pine Drive
Sudbury, MA 01776
978-443-5000
www.jbpub.com
info@jbpub.com

Jones and Bartlett Publishers Canada
2406 Nikanna Road
Mississauga, ON L5C 2W6
CANADA

Jones and Bartlett Publishers International
Barb House, Barb Mews
London W6 7PA
UK

The views expressed in this publication represent the views of the authors and do not necessarily reflect the official views of the National League for Nursing.

ISBN 0-7637-1277-9

This title is a rerelease of a volume originally published in 1994.
ISBN: 0-88737-620-7; Pub. No. 14-2626

Cover art entitled "Family Tree," by Susan Kattas.

Cover design by Lauren Stevens

Multiple quotes excerpted from *The I that is We* by Richard Moss. Copyright ©1981 by Richard Moss. Used by permission of Celestial Arts, Berkeley, CA.

Printed in the United States of America
06 05 04 03 02   10 9 8 7 6 5 4 3 2

IN MEMORY OF

MY MOTHER

Mamie Love Donald Newman

who taught me
to dance and make music
and in the experience of her illness
to let go
live in the present
and love

AND

MY FATHER

Ivo Mathias Newman

who helped me experience
the fun of numbers
the neatness of logic
and the company of contemplation

Acknowledgments

*I*n 1978, when I first presented my ideas on health, someone asked if I would have come to that point in my thinking if I had not been a nurse. It was a question to ponder. I felt like the answer was "Yes," but there was no way of reconstructing the pattern of its coming together. My experience in nursing and the good friends, teachers, colleagues, and students I have known along the way comprise the unique pattern that has unfolded. Joanne Marchione encouraged me to write the first edition—I wasn't sure I had enough to say, but the prospect of doing it was exciting and I told her I would if she would help me, and she did. I want to thank all those who have taken the time to give me feedback on the first edition, particularly Marie Winn and Susan Kattas for their thorough commentaries. I appreciate also Sue Hartman's help in trying to make two-dimensional drawings illustrate the dimensions beyond.

About The Cover

Susan Kattas, MA, the artist of "Family Tree," resides in Hudson, Wisconsin. She uses a pouring technique that invites a dialogue between herself and the painting, a process that she likens to the life process. She identifies with current views arising from physics and Eastern philosophy on the constant interplay of unseen patterns, the interconnectedness of the universe, and the choices human beings have in the cosmic dance. Ms. Kattas acknowledges the parallels of the expansion of her personal journey with the evolving pattern of the whole depicted in Margaret Newman's theory of health as expanding consciousness.

Life has to be in the moment,
spontaneous and vulnerable.
There isn't any winning or losing.
Life itself . . . is the reward
and isn't always easy or fun . . .
the issue of happiness is irrelevant.
The relevant quest is the
expansion of consciousness.

Richard Moss
The I that is We

Contents

Acknowledgments vii

Preface to the Second Edition xv

Introduction xxi

Chapter One Paradigms of Health 1

Chapter Two Pattern of the Whole 15

Chapter Three Theory Underlying Expanding Consciousness 31

Chapter Four Manifestations of Expanding Consciousness .. 49

Chapter Five The Nature of Pattern 69

Chapter Six A Paradigm of Nursing Science 79

Chapter Seven Practice: Order Out of Chaos 95

Chapter Eight From Old Paradigm to New 117

Chapter Nine Letting Go, Moving On 135

Epilogue: A Dialogue with John Heron 143

Appendix: Protocol for Research on Health as Expanding
Consciousness 147

Bibliography 149

Index 165

Preface to the Second Edition

I now realize more fully that the theory of health as expanding consciousness is a radical departure from traditional concepts of health. When I first presented it at a nursing theory conference in New York (Newman, 1978), it had just come together for me—the basic assumptions, the key concepts and their relatedness, the critical insight regarding the wholeness of the evolving pattern. I was aware, as I presented these ideas to that large audience of nurses, that this was something different. There was a quiet stillness and expectancy in the audience. And when I finished, closing with "The responsibility of the nurse is not to make people well, or to prevent their getting sick, but to assist people to recognize the power that is within them to move to higher levels of consciousness," the response was thunderous. It was a turning point. The nurses in that audience in the interactive power of that moment resonated with the meaning of my words. I didn't realize at the time that I was calling for a revolution.

But the essence of the theory required a 180-degree turn. The idea of health held dear to most health professionals was being pushed aside in favor of an idea that incorporated disease as a meaningful manifestation of the whole.

> A really new and radical theory is never just an addition or increment to the existing knowledge. It changes basic rules, requires drastic revision or reformulation of the fundamental assumptions of prior theory, and involves re-evaluation of the existing facts and observations. (Grof, 1985, p. 6)

Diagnosis and treatment of disease were being left to medical science and practice. Recognition of the pattern of the whole was pinpointed as the responsibility of nursing science and practice. This was not an easy shift to make. It could not be explained by reliance on cause-and-effect logic. It was not predictable. It *could* be seen retrospectively in the unfolding of life patterns. It could be experienced in the immediacy of the moment in insight regarding pattern. It is an emergent phenomenon. It makes a difference in the meaning of people's lives.

My early research placed an emphasis on separation of the concepts and control of the environment. This automatic alignment with the traditional scientific method yielded some insights regarding time as an index of consciousness and aging as a process of expanding consciousness but was not sufficiently in tune with the emergent reality of the theory to grasp the dynamic quality of the meaning of the theory for people's lives. As I sought to understand pattern, I gradually moved away from controlled, objective methods to a hermeneutic, dialectic approach. The theory came to life in the research, which I now see as praxis, since it both illuminates the theory and is the essence of practice.

One of the difficulties people have had with the theory of health as expanding consciousness is this: if it is true, it is going to occur naturally. What then is the role of the nurse? In studying pattern recognition, I have become convinced that an important factor in patterning is the mutuality of the presence of someone (a nurse) who has been transformed by the theory with the person(s) being served. In such cases, the interpenetration of the fields of the nurse and client facilitates the transformative process for the client. Bentov once said, "You catch it (expanding consciousness) like you catch the flu." Being imbued with the vision of the theory makes a difference in one's practice.

The actualization of nursing as a learned profession has come a long way since 1985, when I was writing the first edition. Then I searched in vain in the yellow pages and elsewhere to find signs of life of nursing as an independent practicing profession. Now the signs are all around. The nurse case management movement was taking off about that time, especially under the leadership of Phyllis Ethridge, Cathy Michaels, and Gerri Lamb, at Carondelet St. Mary's, in Tucson, a place that has become a national and international center for nurse case management. My ongoing dialogue with these nurses convinces me that we finally (or again) have a model that allows the freedom of theory-guided practice. As health care reform occurs in the United States and abroad, nurses are taking their rightful place in serving society's health care needs.

We also have a much clearer view of the discipline of nursing than we did in 1985. The visions of nursing leaders of over a century have coalesced. The contributions of major nursing thinkers, from Nightingale to the present, have seemed to merge, focusing on two major concepts: health and caring, as interrelated phenomena. The merging of the two concepts seemed, to my colleagues, Marilyn Sime and Sheila Corcoran-

Perry, and me, to be expressed in the phrase: caring in the human health experience. The paradigm of nursing science heralded by Martha Rogers' theory of unitary human beings is integral to that focus. This paradigm specifies that the human being is unitary, that is, cannot be divided into parts, and is inseparable from the larger unitary field. Change takes place in a transformative manner, all-at-once rather than in linear fashion (Newman, Sime, & Corcoran-Perry, 1991; Parse, 1987; Rogers, 1970; Sarter, 1988). The methods of our research have changed considerably to reflect this unitary, transformative perspective.

Research as praxis has come into focus. In nursing's efforts to establish itself in the scientific arena, we devoted a great deal of time and effort to meeting the criteria established by and expected of "hard" scientists. Now with a more complete understanding of the nature of the nursing phenomenon and the emerging clarity of the prevailing paradigm, we can honor the praxis nature of our research. Praxis research is acutely relevant and brings about change in practice immediately. It has allowed my work as a nurse-theorist-researcher to unfold as an undivided whole. I am having more fun.

And we are finally recognizing that a difference in education corresponds to a difference in practice—a difference in the nature, not the value, of the practice. I still have doubts about the extent to which we submit to the hegemony of the medical regime in models of practice that incorporate acute care, but I will offer my perspective on differentiated practice that incorporates instrumental tasks of medical technology.

Many changes, therefore, have taken place since the publication of the first edition of this book. I have tried to make the content congruent with my most recent conceptualizations of theory, research, and practice, but I have left some sections as they were because they represent ideas that have not been fully integrated into our thinking and merit further consideration. I have omitted some of the literature review based on old paradigm views. To update it would be at best tangential to the focus of our discipline. It is clear to me now that the focus of our discipline is the unitary field that combines person-family-community all at once. It is not, as we have argued in the past, individual vis-à-vis family vis-à-vis community nursing, and vice versa. These are false dichotomies based *not* on the discipline of nursing but on previous alignment with medical specialization (including preventive medicine). The focus of medicine *is* the individual, the individual's disease, and secondarily its relationship to the environment. The focus of nursing is the *pattern of the whole*, health as pattern of the evolving whole, with caring as a moral imperative. As we concentrate on this discipline, our practice and the lives of those we serve will be transformed.

M.A.N.
February, 1994

Introduction

*I*ntuition plays a large part in my life. The books I have chosen to read, the people I meet, the jobs I have taken, the places where I live somehow fit together in a pattern that is right for me. Sometimes I have been able to sense the pattern well in advance of its coming together. Other times I just plunge ahead because it feels right. Even seeming mistakes turn out all right in the long run, once you realize there is no such thing as a mistake. Every experience of life is a gift, to be claimed and learned from.

I learned early in life (each time I think of the first instance, I recall an even earlier instance) that events do not always turn out the way you want them to, and that you have a choice: you can be miserable because of it, or you can find a way to make a disagreeable experience meaningful and even enjoyable for you. I decided to pursue the latter.

The most pronounced of these experiences was my mother's nine-year struggle with amyotrophic lateral sclerosis, a degenerative disease of the motor neurons. Her early symptoms began as I was finishing high school and progressed to her partial incapacitation during the years I was away at college, almost unnoticed by me as I was struggling to establish my identity as a young adult. However, once I was back home after college graduation, I was confronted with the unmistake-able dependence of my mother on my brother and sister-in-law and me. I won't go into the details of the professional help we did and did not have, or the agony of the decisions we had to make and the frustration of the infringement on our lives that my mother's illness made. What I do want to share is my realization that life had to be lived in the present, and that if one were to be happy, it had to come one day at a time. I learned that my mother, though physically incapacitated, was a *whole* person, just like anybody else. I came to know her and to love her in a way I probably never would have taken the time to experience had she not been physically depen-dent. The five years I spent with her before she died were difficult, tiring, restrictive in some ways, but intense, loving, and expanding in other ways. As another person has de-scribed it, I have faced great difficulty and have come through it. I had the feeling then that I was preparing for something else.

I had been feeling a call to nursing as a career for a number of years. When I went off to Baylor, a Southern Baptist uni-versity, in 1950, I had no idea what direction my life would take. I was caught up in the religious fervor of my surround-ings for several years and, true to the predominant values of the early fifties, I thought the ideal goal for my life was to be a conscientious and devoted wife. During my junior year, a gnawing conscience-like feeling began to haunt me and never left me alone for very long after that: the feeling that I should become a nurse. There couldn't have been a worse prospect as far as I was concerned! Nursing represented all the things I did not like: illness, hospitals, needles, and so on. The things

I did like, however—math, music, art, dance—did not seem to lead the way to a career for me.

When my mother died, I had just uttered a prayer of willingness to follow that lingering call to nursing. Within two weeks I was enrolled at the University of Tennessee School of Nursing in Memphis.

I knew, after only a few classes, that nursing was right for me. Contrary to my earlier projections, it focused on the complexity of human beings in health and illness, something I had experienced with my mother, and I realized that it was going to demand the best of my intellect as well as the utmost of my humanness. Upon graduation I went almost directly into graduate study, and under the tutelage of a very sensitive, intelligent teacher began to articulate a synthesis of my previous experience and learnings in terms of the essence of the experience of illness and what nursing had to offer.

Basic among these learnings was that illness reflected the life pattern of the person and that what was needed was the recognition of that pattern and acceptance of it for what it meant to that person.

Years later, I came to the conclusion that *health is the expansion of consciousness*. It frightens me to think I might have missed that revelation, it is so important to me now. But even my fear is unwarranted because the gist of all that I am saying is that one can trust the evolving pattern, that it is a pattern of evolving, expanding consciousness *regardless* of what form or direction it may take. This realization is such that illness and disease have lost their demoralizing power. I want to share this realization. We are in the wonderful process of expanding consciousness, of things becoming clearer, of moving from "seeing through a glass darkly" to knowing as we are known.

And there is much more. The expansion of consciousness

is unending. In this way we can embrace aging and death. There is peace and meaning in suffering. We are free from all the things we have feared—loss, death, dependency. We can let go of fear.

★ ★ ★

Throughout my career as an acknowledged theorist, I have been involved, if not embroiled, in the controversy of what is science and what is scientific. In order to side-step that issue here, I would like to say at the outset that this book is not about science in the traditional sense, but rather about *meaning*: The meaning of life and of health and of what those of us in the health professions can do about it. Ken Wilber (1983) captured the point in these statements:

> While we will not shun empirical data (that would miss the point), neither will we confine ourselves to empirical data (that would miss the point completely). (p. 33)

> A physician can describe the intricate biochemical processes that constitute your living being: he [sic] can to some extent repair them, cure them of disease, and operate to remove malfunctions. But he cannot then tell you the *meaning* of that life whose every working mechanism he understands. (p. 2)

The meaning of life and health, I submit, will be found in the evolving process of expanding consciousness.

This book is about a different way of viewing health and disease—a new paradigm. It is grounded in my own personal experience but was stimulated by Martha Rogers' insistence on the unitary nature of a human being in interaction with the environment (Rogers, 1970). While a student in Martha's seminar, I was intrigued, and frustrated, by her statement that health and illness are "simply" expressions of the life process—one no more important than the other. How could that be? Well, possibly they are opposite ends of a continuum. No, she said. How about opposite sides of a coin? No, she said.

So I continued to struggle with this idea until a few years later in a conference with a graduate student about rhythmic phenomena, I had an "Aha" that revealed health and illness as a unitary process, and like rhythmic phenomena, becoming manifest in ups and downs, or peaks and troughs, moving through varying degrees of organization and disorganization, but all as one unitary process. Later my previous introduction to the antagonistic but complementary forces of order and disorder, so essential to our continuing development as self-organizing creatures, became more understandable within the context of health and disease.

Then I became acquainted with Itzhak Bentov's work, which provided logical explanations for many things I had taken on faith up to that point (Bentov, 1978). For instance, Teilhard de Chardin's belief that a person's consciousness continues to develop beyond the physical life and becomes a part of a universal consciousness had made sense to me (Teilhard de Chardin, 1965). Not only was it consistent with my Christian belief of life after death, but it just seemed reasonable that one would not spend a lifetime developing the knowledge and wisdom of one's total being (consciousness) and then have it dissipate into nothing. It made more sense that it continue to develop as part of a larger consciousness.

Bentov's explanations of the evolution of consciousness were matter-of-fact, logical and down to earth. I had the opportunity to hear Bentov speak and to participate in a workshop he led about that time, and I was convinced that this spontaneous, unassuming man *knew* what he was talking about. When accused of talking about religion, he replied, "No, I'm talking about knowledge." When asked how he knew these things, he said, "I just know." What he said felt right. There comes a time when one seeks knowledge that is more than the observable facts.

David Bohm's theory of implicate order helped me to put these thoughts and experiences into perspective (Bohm, 1980). I began to comprehend the underlying, unseen pattern that manifests itself in varying forms, including disease, and the innerconnectedness and omnipresence of all that there is.

Arthur Young's theory of human evolution pinpointed the crucial role of insight, or pattern recognition, and concomitant choice (Young, 1976a, 1976b) and was the impetus for my efforts to integrate the basic concepts of my theory—movement, space, and time, as manifestations of consciousness—into a dynamic portrayal of life and health. Richard Moss's experience of love as the highest level of consciousness (Moss, 1981) provided affirmation and elaboration of my intuition regarding the nature of health and nursing.

As I sit here in awe and feel inadequate to the task of synthesizing these ideas in a meaningful way, I wonder how I could feel otherwise.

Chapter One

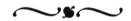

Paradigms of Health

The view of health as the absence of disease has pervaded most of our thinking from very early in life. From the immunizations that prevent devastating childhood diseases to admonitions to brush our teeth and drink our milk, the predominant view is that health (absence of disease) is within our control, and it is our responsibility to make sure we have it. This view is so strong that those who don't have it are viewed as inferior or even repulsive and don't belong with the responsible majority who have exercised the appropriate self-control with its concomitant (or so they think) perfect health. Indeed those who are labeled with a serious disease often question what they have done to deserve this fate or worry about whether or not their family will be able to continue to accept them in their diseased state.

The way we talk about health one would think it is a commodity that can be purchased. We say we can promote it and deliver it. We advise everyone to make sure they have it or get it, because apparently it is possible to lose it. We criticize those who do things that we consider destructive to it, and we even go so far as to disassociate ourselves from them.

We have become idolatrous of health. We have created places of worship of health at which we carry out the recommended rituals to obtain or maintain health. Then when one of the leading gurus dies while engaging in one of these rituals, we say in its defense, "How much sooner would he have died if he had not engaged in it." As if death were the antithesis of health, or the ultimate put-down.

There have been many attempts to get away from the notion of health as the absence of disease. Dunn (1959) was perhaps the first to use the term high-level wellness and portrayed health on a continuum from wellness to illness. Later he defined health as "an integrated method of functioning . . . oriented toward maximizing the potential of which the individual is capable" (Dunn, 1973, p. 7). Dubos (1965), another health spokesman of the sixties, characterized health as the adaptive potential of an individual. He was referring primarily to adaptation to environmental challenges. Others have viewed health in terms of coherence, life style, normality, conformity to social norms, and harmony (Antonovsky, 1979; Ardell, 1977; Dolfman, 1974; Parsons, 1958; Watson, 1985).

Although the authors of these concepts tend to reject the idea of health as the absence of disease, a prevailing notion throughout the health literature is the seeking and accomplishment of a disease-free state. A well-known contemporary, Lewis Thomas (1979), was probably the most explicit in this respect and was convinced that a disease-free state will eventually be accomplished through the work of medical scientists. A featured article based on genetic engineering in a Sunday newspaper magazine section set forth the claim, "Scientists explore the promise of tomorrow—a world without disease" (Ubell, 1985).

The prevailing views of health, then, might be portrayed on a continuum as illustrated below:

DISEASE	ADAPTATION TO DISEASE	ABSENCE OF DISEASE	HIGH LEVEL WELLNESS
ILLNESS $\ominus$			HEALTH $\oplus$

This conceptualization dichotomizes health and illness. Health is the positive state to be desired. Illness (disease) is the negative state. Even though many of the high-level wellness theorists speak of health and illness as integrated, dynamic concepts, a polarization is maintained as one strives for the positive state identified with health and avoids the negative state identified with disease. Disease has been regarded as the *enemy*, that may strike anywhere at any time. The person who is stricken is the *victim*. The troops that *fight* disease are led by the medical *armament*. These commonly used metaphors are illustrative of the way in which our language reinforces disease as the enemy to be overcome and as an entity separate from ourselves. A radical change in our point of view is needed in order to eliminate the dichotomizing of health and disease that has been so prevalent.

A NEW PARADIGM OF HEALTH

There is another view. For a number of years I have been saying that disease is a manifestation of health. This view requires another approach. Certainly we no longer would say we want to promote it or deliver it. On the contrary, we spend a great deal of time and energy trying to prevent disease or get rid of it when it occurs.

Viewing disease as a manifestation of health is a revolutionary idea. The term revolutionary means a sudden, radical, or complete change; a rotation, or about-face; a turning point. To view disease as health, one has to reject a dichotomous or polarized view of health and disease. For those of us accustomed to thinking of these concepts as separate, it helps to apply Hegel's dialectical fusion of opposites and think in terms of a synthesized view: One point of view fuses with the opposite point of view and brings forth a new, synthesized view. In this case, DISEASE fuses with its opposite, absence of disease, NON-DISEASE, and brings forth a new concept of HEALTH:

$$DISEASE—NON\text{-}DISEASE \rightarrow HEALTH$$

This synthesized view incorporates disease as a meaningful aspect of health. Jantsch (1980) goes further and asserts that process thinking transcends a synthesis of opposites, leaving only complementarity, in which the opposites include each other. This would mean that health includes disease, *and* disease includes health. Both of these ways of thinking are echoed by Bohm (1981):

> When you trace a particular absolute notion to what appears to be its logical conclusion, you find it to be identical with its opposite, and therefore the whole dualism collapses, as Hegel found. Reason first shows you that opposites pass into each other, then you discover that one opposite reflects the other, and finally you find that they are identical to each other—not really different at all. (p. 31)

Whichever way one chooses to look at it, the important consideration is that disease is a meaningful reflection of the whole.

Rogers' conceptualization of a person as a unitary being eliminated the usual dichotomy between health and disease (Rogers, 1970). She pointed out that health and illness should be viewed equally as expressions of the life process and that the meaning of these phenomena is derived from an understanding of the life process in its totality. Early critics of Rogers maintained that such a view was unscientific; however an increasingly large number of scientists and philosophers have recognized the limitations of the traditional scientific approach, especially as it relates to the life process and health of human beings, and are calling for an experiential, intuitive recognition of the total patterning of a person.

One of the difficulties in relinquishing a dichotomous view of health and disease is our fragmentary way of thinking and talking. It is easy for us to think of disease separately from health and to proceed to attend to it as a separate part. Dividing things into parts is useful, but eventually becomes more than just a way of thinking about things: It becomes reality itself. We begin to think of disease as really separate from the person it occupies and from the world within and around the person. Our language reinforces this separatism and promotes the idea that one object can act on another object, such as a virus acting on a person, or at best, that objects interact with each other . . . still with the idea of each being a separate, independent entity. This view is no longer sufficient to explain the reality of our world.

Science is demanding a non-fragmentary world view. Experiments at the particle level demonstrate that two particles separated in space display correlated movements simultaneously, indicating "that the various particles have to be taken literally as projections of a higher-dimensional reality which cannot be accounted for in terms of any force of interaction between them" (Bohm, 1980, pp. 186–187). To illustrate, David Bohm suggests envisioning projections of two television cameras (A and B) focused on the same phenomenon from different angles.

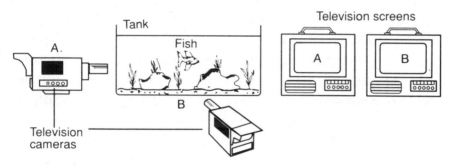

Figure 1.1   Reprinted with permission from Bohm, D. (1980). *Wholeness and the Implicate Order*. London: Routledge & Kegan Paul, p. 187.

Projection A and Projection B contain images that move at the same time and are somehow related, but there is no force of interaction between the two projections and neither portrays the whole picture. Rather, they are manifestations in two-dimensional form of a phenomenon of greater dimensions. The two projections are different points of view of the same larger reality.

Now think of the ways in which we have separated projections of mental phenomena from physical phenomena and substitute Mind and Body for Projections A and B (See Figure 1.2).

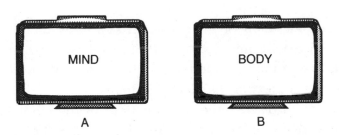

Figure 1.2

Using this analogy, we can see that mind and body are not separate interactive phenomena, but manifestations of the same larger reality. Contrary to previous thinking, one does not cause the other or control the other, as in "mind over matter" terminology, but each is a reflection of an underlying pattern of a phenomenon of greater dimensions. Each is reflective of the larger whole.

   Take this point of view a step further. Substitute Disease and Non-Disease for Projections A and B.

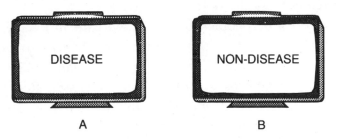

Figure 1.3

Disease and non-disease are not separate entities but *are each reflections of the larger whole*, a phenomenon of greater dimensions.

Reconsideration of the projected synthesis of health and disease reveals a new concept: PATTERN OF THE WHOLE. This is the primary, underlying, indivisible pattern which includes the context of the identified focus.

This point of view (health as pattern of the whole) is consistent with Bohm's theory of implicate order (Bohm, 1980). According to Bohm, there exists in our universe an unseen, multidimensional pattern that is the ground, or basis, for all things. This is the implicate order. Arising out of the implicate order is the explicate order, a kind of precipitate of the implicate order. The explicate order includes the tangibles of our world. These tangibles, the things we can see, touch, hear, feel, are so much more real to us than the underlying unseen pattern that we think the explicate order is primary—the real thing. Actually, according to Bohm, the implicate order is primary. The explicate order arises periodically from the implicate, like waves appearing and disappearing on the surface of the ocean. The explicate, whatever form it may take, is a temporary manifestation of a total undivided pattern, which Bohm refers to as the holomovement.

A number of people concerned with health have recognized the failure of a frontal attack on disease in bringing about significant changes in our sense of health and well being (Capra, 1982; Dossey, 1982; Pelletier, 1985). Relating the efforts of modern medicine to Bohm's theory of implicate order, Dossey (1982) stated:

> They focus only on the reality of the explicate order, the realm of our habitation, where the world is one of separate objects and events. The implicate domain, where the very meaning of health, disease, and death radically changes, is currently of no concern to medicine. (p. 189)

In the context of the theory of implicate order, *manifest health, encompassing disease and non-disease, can be regarded as the explication of the underlying pattern of person-environment.* Common observable phenomena—such as body temperature, blood pressure and heart rate; neoplasms and biochemical variations; immune reactions; diet and exercise; communication; family relations; environmental pollution—are explicate manifestations of the pattern of the whole. Viewing these manifestations as reflections of the underlying, dynamic pattern makes it possible for us to *see* the pattern of the whole and thereby begin to understand it.

The theory of biological rhythms is helpful in seeing health and illness as a unitary process, a fluctuating pattern of rhythmic phenomena. There are times when the pattern of a person becomes increasingly disorganized, similar to when one's physiological rhythms are out of phase. This situation can continue until the person becomes what we ordinarily regard as "sick." The sickness then can provide a kind of shock that reorganizes the relationships of the person's pattern in a more harmonious way. Consider the function of a high fever, or an emotional crisis, or the accident that occurs at a particularly crucial time. These, and other critical incidents, may provide the shock that facilitates a jump from one pattern to another, presumably at a higher level of organization. So, if we view disease as something discrete, something to be avoided, diminished, or eliminated altogether, we may be ruling out the very factor that can bring about the unfolding of the life process that the person is naturally seeking. Illness may accomplish for people what they secretly want but are not able to acknowledge even to themselves. Ferguson (1980) pointed out that people who get sick don't want to be their "old self" again; she described a woman who had had a stroke and who "conceded that she hadn't faced the fact that she wanted to change her life. So the stroke changed her life" (p. 252).

THE PARADIGM SHIFT

Ferguson (1980) outlined the paradigm shift taking place in regard to health. Several of the changes are particularly relevant to the point being made here that disease is a meaningful aspect of health. The shift is from treatment of symptoms to a search for *patterns*; from viewing pain and disease as wholly negative to a view that pain and disease are *information*; from seeing the body as a machine in good or bad repair to seeing the body as a *dynamic field of energy* continuous with the larger field; from seeing disease as an entity to seeing it as a *process*.

This paradigm shift is apparent in the nursing literature. The conceptual models that originated in the 1950s and '60s were based on a view of the patient as a person in good or bad repair and needing more or less help from nursing to regain or attain a state referred to as maximum health or well being. Rogers' conceptualization of person-environment represented a turning point (Rogers, 1970). The absence of boundaries between person and environment and the emphasis on mutual simultaneous interaction of person-environment demanded a non-dichotomous view. Rogers' insistence on a unitary view of the pattern of person-environment demanded a view of the person as an emerging pattern of the whole.

The old paradigm of health, based on the medical model, recognizes separate parts and advocates an instrumental approach. One identifies what is wrong in a system and tries to fix it.

The new paradigm of health, essential to nursing, embraces a unitary pattern of changing relationships. It is developmental (Newman, 1992a). The task is not to try to change another person's pattern but to recognize it as information that depicts the whole and relate to it as it unfolds.

The instrumental paradigm is linear, causal, predictive, dichotomous, rational, and controlling. The relational paradigm is patterned, emergent, unpredictable, unitary, intuitive, and innovative. The new paradigm incorporates the old paradigm and transforms it. When Copernicus introduced the view of the universe with the sun, rather than the earth, as the center, his view retained the phenomena of the old view but explained them from a different standpoint. The shift in paradigms from Newtonian physics to Einsteinian and further to quantum theory presents a broader, more complete explanation of phenomena but reaffirms the old relationships under certain conditions. Therefore, it is important to think of the characteristics of the old paradigm of health as special cases of the new. Viewed within the context of pattern, information from the old paradigm will have new meaning.

Chapter Two

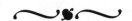

Pattern of the Whole

To see health as the pattern of the whole, we need to see disease not as a separate entity that invades our bodies but as a manifestation of the evolving pattern of person-environment interaction. The pattern being signalled by disease (as well as non-disease) can be seen and understood in terms of a pattern of energy. Physical illness or intense emotional activity may be regarded as manifestations of blocked energy beyond our awareness (Moss, 1981, p. 80). Although we cannot always "see" energy, we accept that it is a characteristic of the human field. Disease makes it possible for us to envision a general pattern of the energy flow of a person. For example, hypertension may connote a pattern of contained (pressured) energy, hyperthyroidism a pattern of diffuse, multidirectional energy, or diabetes the inability to use available energy. Each of these patterns vary, of course, according to the unique configuration of each person-environment situation. The disease can be regarded as a manifestation of pattern and can assist people in becoming aware of their pattern of interacting with the environment.

The following story illustrates this point. A number of

17

years ago a friend of mine was diagnosed as having hyperthyroidism and was being treated by a leading endocrinolo-
gist. She had been on medication for approximately a year
with very little progress in alleviating the disease. The endo-
crinologist had indicated that she probably would have to
have surgery to have the thyroid gland removed. But before
she pursued that alternative she went to see Dora Kunz, a
sensitive person who has the ability to see (in terms of energy
flow) the patterns of people's interactions as they relate to
their diseases (Weber, 1984). As my friend related to me the
things Dora had told her, this is what I gleaned from it: That
Dora could visualize her energy being diffused in every direction (in a slightly diminished intensity probably because of the
medications she was taking to reduce the activity of the thyroid gland). Dora concluded that it was not relevant to tell my
friend to curtail her activities in order to conserve her energy.
The pattern of intense multidirectional energy expenditure
was her way of life. The only thing Dora could suggest for my
friend was that she make sure she took in enough energy to
sustain her way of life.

To fill in some of the details of my friend's life, she was the
oldest of nine children and was looked to for advice and assistance not only by her siblings but also by her parents. She was
a member of a religious community of nuns and freely ful-
filled her responsibilities to other members of the community
during their frequent visits. She was a faculty member in a
large urban university and enthusiastically carried more than
her share of teaching responsibilities along with a larger-than-
usual number of committee responsibilities. She could rarely
say "No" to any request. She was a caring friend to many
people—typically staying up half the night to bake a birthday
cake or do some similar favor.

Dora's picture of her energy going in many directions was reflective of her life. And it was accurate that she was not taking in enough energy to sustain that way of life—not taking time to sleep or eat or rest. When I really began to think about it, her thyroid gland was trying to produce the energy she needed. The medical/surgical approach to diminish or delete the activity of the thyroid gland was just the opposite of what her system was trying to accomplish.

My friend did begin to pay more attention to her energy intake and did not have to have surgery and even was able to eliminate or greatly reduce the medications she was taking. *But I do not want to imply that simply balancing her energy intake-output did the trick.* I surmise that the transforming factor was the *insight* she gained regarding her own pattern of life. This is the understanding that Young (1976b) referred to as accelerating the evolution of consciousness. And perhaps, as has already been suggested, she discovered herself in this pattern, found peace in the congruity, and was able to move to a higher level of organization and harmony. Moss (1981) stated:

> We must attain higher energy states to begin to transmute the reality that appears unchangeable at our present energy level. Whether this occurs through the spontaneous awakening of energies or through a disease process is of little importance. (p. 101)

The pattern of a person that eventually manifests itself as disease is primary. The disease is a manifestation of the underlying pattern. This point is germane to Chinese medicine (Tiller, 1973) and has been illustrated in plants by Kirlian photography (Ostrander & Schroeder, 1971). Ravitz's early work correlating bioelectrical potentials with disease indicated that the change in the bioelectrical field preceded subjective and behavioral changes associated with illness (Ravitz, 1962).

Profiles of interactive patterns that correlate with disease states, especially coronary heart disease and cancer, have been described in the literature for at least a quarter of a century. My research, and that of my colleagues, has sought to elaborate the pattern of persons with these and other major medical problems as manifestations of the pattern of the whole (Jonsdottir, *in progress*; Lamendola & Newman, 1994; Moch, 1990; Newman & Moch, 1991). Themes for each category of participants have generally supported the profiles from previous research and are illustrative of the pattern of disease as pattern of the whole. These general profiles, however, are insufficient in addressing the individuality of the pattern demanded by the unitary-transformative paradigm of nursing science and practice. The unitary-transformative perspective becomes evident in the unique pattern of each individual person-environment trajectory.

DISEASE AS INTEGRATING FACTOR

It seems strange to say (strange because it's part of the revolutionary shift) but disease may be the way a person gets in touch with his or her pattern. Many of us have lived our lives in such a way that we have not become fully aware of ourselves or our own pattern. The pattern may then manifest itself in a more "unconscious" manner, in terms of changes that may be interpreted as maladaptive, or disease, but which may represent movement to a higher level of consciousness. Certain forms of psychosis may be an indication of a person's involvement in an important personal transformation (Pelletier, 1978). Physical disease may serve the same purpose—

even more so—since physical changes associated with inter-nalization of stress may represent a person's inability to be fully aware of stress. Moss (1981) related that "what may un-fold unconsciously at one level of consciousness and finally present as disease may now be perceived as an energetic shift which becomes an unfolding process" (p. 75). This relates to Moss's position that some of what is labeled disease might be considered stalled or overly rapid penetrations of higher ener-gies. This is similar to Rogers' position that some of our dis-eases are manifestations of evolutionary emergence of higher energy states. According to Moss, our individual behaviors [diseases?] describe "what we don't dissolve into" (how we separate ourselves). It takes energy to maintain the me that is separate and this may translate into disease.

Disease may be considered an integrating factor (Stone, 1978), and as such, is important in the evolutionary develop-ment of the person. Evolution thrives on tension (Watson, 1978). Contrary to what one might think, disequilibrium is im-portant in maintaining active exchange with the environment (Jantsch, 1980), and active exchange with the environment is essential for growth (Land, 1973). The tension characteristic of disease may provide an important disequilibriant in the growth process, and therefore, may be regarded as a facilita-tor of that process. We evolve by having our own equilibrium thrown off balance and then discovering how to attain a new state of balance, temporarily, and then moving on to another phase of disequilibrium. This is a natural process, according to Fuller (1975):

"The forces of the field of energy . . . interoscillate through the symmetry of equilibrium to various asymmetries, never paus-ing at equilibrium. The vector equilibrium itself is only a referential pattern of conceptual relationships at which nature never pauses" (p. 27).

Dossey (1982) agreed and viewed disease as a natural perturbation that offers human beings the chance to evolve to a new and higher level of complexity.

DISEASE AS AN EMERGENT PATTERN

For years Martha Rogers has considered various diseases as emergent patterns. More recently cultural historian William Irwin Thompson, systems theorist Will McWhinney, and musician David Dunn have declared the HIV/AIDS phenomenon as a signal of the emergence of a new culture. They regarded the loss of membranal integrity characteristic of AIDS as similar to the breaking down of boundaries at a global level, as seen in geographical changes and diminishing ideological differences. Thompson (1989) characterized the HIV not as an object but as a herald of the need to live together in symbiotic relationships:

> We may need to change our ideas of treatment to ones in which the immune system is "retuned" to new states of harmonic integration in which we learn to tolerate aliens by seeing the self as a cloud in a clouded sky and not as a lord in a walled-in fortress. (p. 99)

Within this theoretical context a study of the evolving patterns of persons with HIV/AIDS was conducted (Lamendola & Newman, 1994) and revealed patterns consistent with the theory of expanding consciousness. The men "moved from being separated, alienated individuals in search of their place and connection in life to more meaningful, authentic relationships with self and others" (p. 9).

DISEASE AS EXPANDING CONSCIOUSNESS

The process of life is toward higher levels of consciousness. Sometimes this process is smooth, pleasant, harmonious; other times it is difficult, disharmonious, as in disease. Moss (1981) wrote:

> I believe that, when the new level of energy is attained, the forces that might have configured disease at the old level no longer need operate. If it is not attained, then the disease probably perseveres and physical death may become the transformative door. In either case, transformation of consciousness has occurred, and to a deeper level of our Beingness this may be all that really matters. (p. 101)

The conclusions of Lerner and Remen (1985), based on their work with cancer patients, support this view:

> But what is most striking to me about many of these people with cancer has nothing to do with evidence of extended disease-free intervals or life expectancy. What amazes and touches me is that through this difficult life passage they have found inner resources of strength, wisdom, and insight that they often had not experienced before. They do not live with certainties of clear victories. They live with the knowledge that the cancer process may worsen or return at any time, and with the personal conviction that how they live may affect when or whether it does so. But the kind of life they develop is also the one that they would want to follow even if their efforts had no impact on the course of the disease. (p. 32)

Fryback (1993), too, found support for the meaningfulness of disease in people with cancer and AIDS. She found the study participants allowing their lives to unfold in a satisfying, purposeful way.

When we begin to think of ourselves as centers of consciousness (patterns of energy) within an overall pattern of expanding consciousness, we can begin to see that what we sense of our lives is part of a much larger whole. First the pattern of consciousness that is the person; then broadening the focus, the pattern of consciousness that is the family and physical surroundings; then the pattern that is the community, the person's larger environmental affiliations, such as work or school; and ultimately the pattern of the world. It is this pattern of the whole that is the phenomenon of nursing's practice.

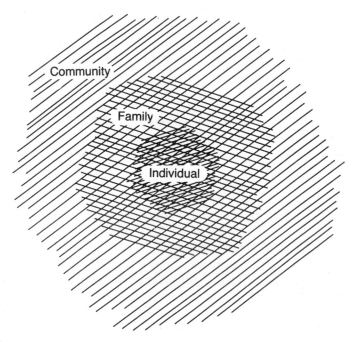

Figure 2.1   Individual-Family-Community as pattern of the whole.

EXTENDING THE PATTERN TO ENCOMPASS FAMILY AND COMMUNITY

We are not separate people with separate diseases. We are open energy systems constantly interacting and evolving with each other. The pattern manifested by a disease does not stop with one person but is part of the greater whole. In the process of considering the pattern of interaction of an individual with the environment, one inevitably considers the pattern of interaction of the family and the community.

A man in South Dakota shared how his father's experience with amyotrophic lateral sclerosis was a transforming process for an entire family. His father, an active man who had overcome polio and residual disability to become a successful businessman and politician, first fought the decline in his abilities brought on by the disease, then later began to accept these limitations. That acceptance was a turning point. The entire family became involved in assisting his father with his daily needs and the endless encounters with the medical system. There were changes in his father: "I saw Dad go from an aggressive, seemingly insensitive man to an accepting, aware, and tender person," and in his mother: "Part of his [Dad's] expanding consciousness, and that of the family, was the excitement and partial ownership he felt in my mother's expanding role and consciousness as a business woman. In three short years she took over the agency, passed each and every state exam and license, and was elected Businesswoman of the Year. You think he didn't play a part in that?" This six-year experience was one of loving intensity and uncertainty and transformation that involved the entire family.

People often ask how it is possible to apply the theory of expanding consciousness to situations in which a child comes into the world with a developmental disability. This story of Aaron, who was severely disabled following fetal distress at birth, illustrates a pattern of expanding consciousness not only for his family but also for the community. It's referred to as "Aaron's legacy" (Tommet, 1992).

Aaron's parents, Jan and Tom, at first experienced the shock and sorrow of realizing that there was something wrong with their newborn child, who had frequent seizures. The first step was to understand what had happened to him and to find out who within the medical profession they could call on for help in this difficult situation. The first six months of Aaron's life was a constant struggle to deal with the complexity and uncertainty of his condition.

Jan was frustrated by Aaron's resistance to her attempts to cuddle him, but with the help of a rehabilitation specialist she began to understand Aaron's resistance to touch as over-stimulation of his sensitive body. Jan spoke of each day as a constant struggle for survival:

> There was no joy in our lives. I felt like constantly treading water to keep our heads afloat.

There was the additional strain of finding someone to care for Aaron, so that Jan and Tom could receive some respite from the constant struggle and, eventually, so that Jan could return to work, something she felt she needed in order to restore some balance in her life.

The Developmental Achievement Center (DAC) was a source of hope and assistance in their desire to enhance the quality of Aaron's life. After the first year, all the critical support systems were in place, except that it was still difficult to establish respite care. They had no extended family in the area and the alternatives they tried were unsatisfactory.

Jan and Tom began to reach out to others. At their suggestion, the DAC started a support group for families facing similar situations. With great fear, they decided to continue to have children. With the help of a high-risk specialist and a nurse for ongoing therapy and monitoring, Jan gave birth to a baby girl, Leah, when Aaron was 2½, and later to a third child, Evan, both of whom were a real joy to the family. Both infants related to Aaron by rolling over him, as he was no longer so sensitive to touch, and lying on him and doing all the physical touching. He was able to respond to the cuddling. He was learning to communicate his needs, and Jan and Tom were able to understand what he wanted. Both Leah and Evan were supportive of Aaron's learning.

Because of Jan's awareness of Aaron's response to Leah and Evan and of their response (in terms of curiosity) to him, Jan worked to establish a program at the public school that integrated children with and without disabilities. She wanted to create more understanding between the two and to prevent Aaron's being isolated from the mainstream of society. The program was established, and even though Aaron never had the chance to participate in it (he died at age 5½), Jan feels that "part of his legacy is that program." Here are Jan's concluding remarks:

> I think that Aaron taught our family a lot about this issue of belonging and being part of a community. Aaron's short life . . . in some ways he was much more powerful than me in being able to facilitate some changes just in attitudes by his presence. And that despite the tragedy and the sorrow of his situation, I value what he gave to us and sometimes I kind of

miss his sense of spirit—which was a driving force for me . . .
it was so intense and so severe that there almost was no
choice. There is a choice—but there is almost like no choice
because you have to do the best you can and more.

In the beginning of the interview, when Jan was asked to tell
about the most meaningful experience in her life, she introduced the above story by saying it was "a very profound experience that changed my life dramatically. I think the reason
it was probably a profound experience was the fact that it
changed me and it changed my relationships with people. It
changed my understanding of the world. The experience that
I'm talking about was Aaron's birth, his whole life and his
death, and . . . what's happened since his death, too, in terms
of a legacy, his legacy. . . . What happened to me was a very
deep, very intimate, very powerful experience."

Jan's experience illustrates graphically the pattern of the
whole as it expanded from the individual to the family to the
community. There were no separate parts.

The premise that illness in one family member is reflected
in the pattern of family interaction was introduced in the
fifties in psychiatry and may be extended within the theory of
health as expanding consciousness to any family situation.
There is no intent to imply causality. The pattern simply *is*.
The disease simply is reflected in the pattern, a pattern of
evolving consciousness of the family. Central to this view is
the premise that disease is an integrative and transformative
factor in the family system.

The pattern of the whole contains the individual as an
open system interacting with the family as an open system
interacting with the community as an open system. The previous assumptions apply also when focusing on the commu-

nity. Health of the community is conceptualized in terms of changing patterns of energy in the evolution of the system. A pattern of disease endemic to a community can be considered a manifestation of the pattern of community health. The holo-movement can be seen in spatial, temporal, and movement patterns that reflect the overall pattern of the community. For example, the areas of the community that are open or closed, and at what times of the day, and whether or not movement flows freely through the community. The diversity and quality of interaction within the community and between the community and its larger environment are indicators of the level of consciousness, and thus of the health, of the community.

IS DISEASE NECESSARY?

It is possible to move to higher levels of consciousness without the necessity of disease. The degree of fluidity with which we interact with stress determines how disabling it will be (Bentov, 1978; Moss, 1981). Openness allows the energies to pass through. This means that we accept the experience as *our* experience regardless of how contrary it is to what we might have wished would happen. If we reject the experience, we reject ourselves and we initiate the process of defending ourselves against ourself (fighting off the offender) and the stress-related physical changes occur. When we let go of personal control (which we don't have anyway), life is de-stressed. This does not mean that we do not act, or that we passively are run over by whatever comes our way. It simply means we accept it and interact with it as *our* experience. We recognize that we are one aspect of a much larger whole that is evolving to a higher order, and learn from the experience. Moss (1981) believes "that all disease and all suffering starts as we begin to recoil away from this deeper intuition of the vastness and indefinable eternity of Self. When the fear or doubt arises, which it does over and over again, it becomes a signal that it is time to let go, rebalance and find an unconditional allowing of life" (p. 29).

Chapter Three

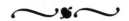

Theory Underlying
Expanding Consciousness

*T*he evolving pattern of person-environment can be viewed as a process of expanding consciousness. The assumption is made that consciousness is coextensive in the universe and is the essence of all matter (Bentov, 1978; Muses, 1978). Persons as individuals, and human beings as a species, are identified by their patterns of consciousness. The person does not *possess* consciousness—the person *is* consciousness.

The key to understanding this view of consciousness is in its definition. Consciousness is defined as the *information* of the system: The capacity of the system to interact with the environment. In the human system the informational capacity includes not only all the things we normally associate with consciousness, such as thinking and feeling, but also all the information embedded in the nervous system, the endocrine system, the immune system, the genetic code, and so on. The information of these and other systems reveals the complexity of the human system and how the information of the system interacts with the information of the environmental system.

The immune system is a good example. It is set up in such a way that when information not recognized by the system enters the system, it produces particles designed specifically to interact with the new information. This kind of information is part of the consciousness of the system. The more highly developed the system, the more complex the informational capacity, and the more varied and numerous the responses to the environment. Jantsch points out that "If consciousness is defined as the degree of autonomy a system gains in the dynamic relations with its environment, even the simplest autopoietic systems . . . have a primitive form of *consciousness*" (Jantsch, 1980, p. 40).

Bentov (1978) depicted the evolution of consciousness as ranging from "inanimate" objects, like rocks, at the lowest end of the range, to astral and spiritual "beings" beyond the human level. Rocks display a low level of consciousness in terms of quantity and quality of interaction with the environment; yet there *is* some interaction, and when one considers the interactional capacity of some crystals, it may be that the consciousness of rocks is much greater than we have imagined. Moving up to plants, animals, and eventually the human being, one can see the increasing complexity of the categories with the concomitant increasing ability to interact with the environment based on the information of the system, e.g., the ability of plants to utilize nutrients from the environment, the variety of response afforded by the mobility of animals, and even more so by the higher cortical abilities of humans. With increases in levels of consciousness, the system forms more intricate nervous systems, capable of interacting with nature in more complex patterns.

There is openness of interaction throughout the entire spectrum of consciousness. The human being interacts with animals and plants on one end of the spectrum and astral and spiritual beings at the other end. All creation is in constant and instantaneous contact.

Our realities are not the same. Reality depends on where one falls within the spectrum of consciousness. When contemplating the range of human consciousness, one can imagine that persons at either end of a normal curve might appear to be abnormal (or pathological?) to others in the middle of the human range. At the upper end there is a greater refinement of response in terms of insight, context and detail (Bentov, 1978).

Bentov compared total, or absolute, consciousness to a boundless deep sea that appears calm and smooth *but contains tremendous energy and is full of creative potential*. It consists of infinitely fine vibration of high frequency, low amplitude waves. As they approach infinity, they approach a straight line of absolute consciousness (Bentov, 1978).

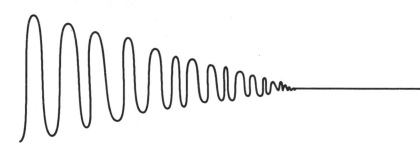

Figure 3.1

Absolute consciousness is "a state in which *contrasting concepts become reconciled and fused. Movement and rest fuse into one*" (Bentov, 1978, p. 67). To extrapolate further, so do love and hate, good and evil. But returning to the metaphor of the ocean, one can see ripples on the surface. This is our manifest, physical reality.

These descriptions by Bentov correspond to Bohm's analogies of the implicate/explicate order. The calm, unruffled sea of creative potential corresponds to the implicate order; the waves of matter correspond to the explicate order. Bentov maintained that all matter is evolving toward higher levels of consciousness. We are on our way, ready or not! Matter *is* the vibrating, changing component of pure consciousness (Bentov, 1978).

This view of matter as the manifestation of consciousness reaffirms the unitary nature of the human being. Mind and matter are made of the same basic stuff. The difference is in the speed and intensity of the energy waves: Mind represents faster, higher energy waves, and matter represents slower, lower energy waves. Bentov offers the analogy of ice and steam: One is solid, the other more diffuse, but both are manifestations of water in different form.

THE EVOLUTION OF NEW FORMS

The creative potential embedded in absolute consciousness, or the implicate order, has a self-organizing capability. The process of evolving to higher levels of consciousness is consistent with Rogers' (1970) assumption of increasing complexity in living systems and is supported by Prigogine's theory of dissipative structures (Prigogine & Stengers, 1984).[1]

Dissipative structures have two complementary aspects: (1) deterministic behavior based on the average values of the variables involved and (2) amplification of the fluctuations of the system leading to a change in structure. A new order appears when a giant fluctuation becomes stabilized by exchange of energy with the environment. It goes like this: The system operates in a rhythmic, predictable fashion for a while until a chance element, some critical event, brings about a giant fluctuation that propels the system into disorganized, unpredictable fluctuations, from which the system will eventually emerge at a higher level of organization.

---

[1]This theory explains the paradox of decreasing order (entropy) in physical processes and increasing order (negative entropy) in living systems (Prigogine, 1980; Prigogine, Allen & Herman, 1977). Entropy is based on observations within a closed system (linear transformations close to equilibrium), one in which energy can enter and leave but mass cannot. Such a system will evolve through irreversible processes to a state of maximum entropy, i.e., maximum disorder. This type of evolution is *not* the basis for the evolution of living systems. Living systems are open systems, i.e., systems undergoing irreversible nonlinear transformation far from equilibrium. These systems are capable of exchanging both energy and matter with the environment. When properties of thermodynamics are extended to open systems, new properties emerge: the capacity for self-organization, i.e., spontaneous shift from lower to higher levels of organizational complexity (Prigogine, Allen & Herman, 1977). A major point is that irreversible processes play a fundamental constructive role.

A local region of the living system is both a positive-entropy (disorder) source that dumps into the environment and a negative-entropy (order) sink which drains negative entropy from the environment so as to increase the internal order and complexity of the local region. Prigogine names such self-organizing systems "dissipative structures," since they maintain their organizational complexity by continually dissipating high entropy energy that they produce back into the environment.

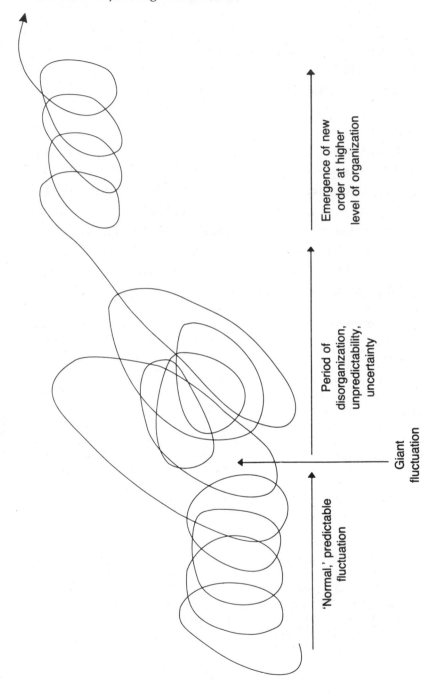

Figure 3.2   The process depicted by Prigogine's theory of dissipative structures.

Then the rhythmic, orderly fluctuation resumes at this higher level (See Figure 3.2). This evolution requires energy from the environment. A single form of species "in competition for resources evolves in such a way that hitherto untapped resources are exploited, and each resource is exploited with increasing effectiveness" (Prigogine, Allen & Herman, 1977, p. 3).

Mishel's reconceptualization of uncertainty in illness, defined as the "inability to determine the meaning . . . or to accurately predict outcomes" (1990, p. 256), corresponds to the period of disorganization of Prigogine's process of dissipative structures. Mishel has expanded the theory of uncertainty to include growth and self-organization as the outcome of coping with uncertainty and incorporates themes that correspond to basic assumptions of the theory of health as expanding consciousness: open systems, increasing complexity, unidirectionality of change over time. Uncertainty is viewed as an opportunity for a person to make a transition during illness from one perspective of life to one at a higher order. This concept of uncertainty is important to the theory of health as expanding consciousness.

The similarities between the functioning of a society and that of dissipative structures is described as follows:

> Firstly, societies have complex non-linear interactions between their elements derived from the cooperation and conflicts involved in the attempts of individuals and groups to attain "goals." Secondly, they are subject to local "behavioral fluctuations," meaning that sometimes new behavior can appear, such as an invention, a modification of group organization, or a new goal or belief, and this can either be suppressed by the social environment or will grow and spread until the society itself is modified. Here again we find the dual aspects of change and determinism, and the theory briefly described here

. . . serve as a background for discussion of the evolution of social systems. (Prigogine, Allen & Herman, 1977, p. 4)

In comparing this theory to their observations of planetary motion, these authors commented: "Instead of finding stability and harmony, wherever we look we discover evolutionary processes leading to diversification and increasing complexity" (pp. 5–6).

Prigogine's theory is based on the fact that all dynamic systems fluctuate, but rather than averaging out, the process itself becomes supraordinate to the random perturbations and shifts to *a new, higher order*, more complex structural form. At this new level of organization, a new set of functional principles apply, and a new order is attained through fluctuation at another level. The richer the resources of the environment, the greater the diversity. The more elements that enter into interaction, the greater the chance of instability, and, therefore, the greater the chance of new traits coming into being (Prigogine, Allen & Herman, 1977).

Sheldrake (1983) also addressed the phenomenon of new forms coming into being. In his hypothesis of formative causation, he stated that characteristic forms and behavior of physical, chemical and biological systems in the present moment are determined by invisible organizing fields acting across time and space. He referred to these fields as morphogenetic fields, which he conceived as being without mass or energy.

Sheldrake cited a 1920 learning experiment on rats conducted by William McDougall. In these experiments, the task remained the same but later generations of rats learned the task more quickly than earlier generations. In subsequent experiments designed to replicate this finding, the first generation learned almost as quickly as McDougall's last generation;

some learned immediately without error. Sheldrake hypothesized that the first generation established a morphogenetic field for the specific behavior being learned and that this field guided the behavior of other generations via morphic resonance.

According to Sheldrake, the effect of the morphogenetic field is not diminished by space or time and is cumulative. This theory lends an explanation to the observed phenomenon that the difficulty of synthesizing new compounds becomes increasingly easier once the compound has been formed the first time, and this facility is apparent in laboratories great distances from each other. *It gives pattern a role in the development and evolution of physical and biological systems.* The activity of the central nervous system can be understood in terms of spatio-temporal patterns of chemical and electrical activity (energy), or as patterns of consciousness.

Whyte (1974), in his final philosophical treatise, spoke of the two great general tendencies of order and disorder and pointed out the fallacy of their *apparent* opposition. Rather he saw them as complementary and indispensable antagonists. He spoke of these tendencies as contrasting coexisting systems, not the clash of opposed principles (Whyte, 1974). Watson (1978) speculated that evolution requires a rival plan, that DNA is joined by a rival program in the mitochondria that sets evolution free from the constraints of the body, from the dictates of the genes. Evolution thrives on instability and tension.

PATTERN RECOGNITION AS TURNING POINT IN THE EVOLUTION OF CONSCIOUSNESS

Understanding of the role of pattern recognition in the process of expanding consciousness is enhanced by Arthur

Young's theory of human evolution (Young, 1976b). Young identified three types of evolution. The first involves the genotype, changes effected by DNA in the design of the mechanism. The second manifests itself as animal instinct, or learned behavior, and begins only when there is the possibility of choice. The third, incorporating the previous two, is possible for human beings; it is the possibility of *understanding* and brings with it much more rapid evolutionary change. This type of evolution is not gradual, as are the previous types, but occurs instantaneously:

> Primarily it is *recognition*, recognition of a principle, realization of a truth, reconciliation of a duality, *satori*. It is at once the privilege of man, and the formative principle that enables man to evolve. (p. 180)

Insight has been equated with pattern recognition (Hart, 1978) and with the inner voice that some people consider their intuition.

Pattern recognition is a turning point in human evolution. Young (1976b) took the position that the evolution of matter represents a fall from total freedom into determinism. From Young's perspective, the stage of determinate matter represents a turning point at which matter takes on one of the characteristics of living systems and is able to utilize energy from the environment in a self-organizing fashion, i.e., the reversal of entropy:

> . . . it is no longer appropriate to think of the universe as a gradually subsiding agitation of billiard balls. The universe, far from being a desert of inert particles, is a theatre of increasingly complex organization, a stage for development in which man has a definite place, and without any upper limit to his evolution. (p. xxiv)

Young designated light as the whole from which the universe has evolved and as the origin of everything, including "the eternal now of consciousness" (p. 28). Movement from light to determinate matter involves increasing loss of freedom (light) or increase in constraints; movement from determinate matter back to the light incorporates corresponding gains in freedom.

Wilber (1981) saw the emergence of the human being's consciousness as separate from the world as a stage of development in which duality existed. The meaning of the developmental process is the transcendence of the separate self into superconsciousness, a return to the wholeness of the Absolute, and with it the end of the tyranny of time.

The testimony of these scientists/philosophers presents some agreement that life is evolving in the direction of higher levels of consciousness; that complementary forces of order and disorder maintain a fluctuating field that periodically transcends itself and shifts into a higher order of functioning; and that in humans this evolutionary process is facilitated by insight and involves a transcendence of the spatial-temporal self to a spiritual realm.

THE EVOLUTION OF CONSCIOUSNESS AS THE PROCESS OF HEALTH

The process of the evolution of consciousness is the process of health. Human beings come from a state of potential consciousness into the world of determinate matter and have the capacity for understanding that enables them to gain insight regarding their patterns. This insight represents a turning point in evolving consciousness with concomitant gains in freedom of action. Young (1976b) regarded the stage of determinate matter as a necessary laboratory for testing one's understanding of the way things work. He saw the life process as a sequence of learning to *use* a "law" rather than be blocked by it. He saw *action* rather than matter as basic.

This task is particularly relevant where disease is concerned. The physical manifestations of disease may be considered evidence of how one is interacting with the environment. In this sense this illustrates the laboratory to which Young refers. The task is to gain an understanding of that pattern and to work with it.

The central theme of Young's theory is that a self, or a universe, is of the same nature. The essential nature is undefinable, but the beginning and the end are characterized by complete freedom, unrestricted choice. The steps in between are a sequence of first, losses of freedom, as identity in the form of a physical being evolves, and then a reversal of these losses as entropy is reversed and understanding evolves.

Young (1976b) described this development as first a loss of freedom and then a reversal of the process as the human being moves toward total freedom:

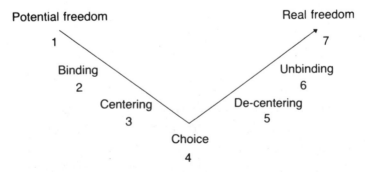

Figure 3.3 Young's spectrum of the evolution of consciousness.

The goal, according to Young, is to reach a higher level of development, and the process is one of interaction of persons with one another and with the social state.

The second stage of Young's model is characterized by binding. The individual is sacrificed for the sake of the collective. Everything is regulated for the individual, and there is no need for initiative. In the third stage, centering, an individual identity is established and along with it self-consciousness and self-determination. Individualism emerges in the self's break with authority.

The fourth stage, choice, is the turning point. The task of the fourth stage is to learn the "law." The emphasis is on science and on searching for laws. It involves a more advanced stage of combination of people and things and an eventual realization that the devices invented are no longer solutions to the situation. Answers to the problems require a different kind of solution from those previously considered "progress." A new awareness of self-limitation precedes inner growth. The turning point is a kind of inward, self-generated reformation.

The fifth stage, de-centering, begins when the "law" is learned. In this stage emphasis shifts from the development of self (individuation) to dedication to something greater than the individual self. The person experiences outstanding competence; their works have a life of their own beyond the creator. The task is the transcendence of the ego. Form is transcended, and energy becomes the dominant feature—in terms of animation, vitality, a quality that is somehow infinite. Pattern is higher than form; the pattern can manifest itself in different forms. In this stage the person experiences the power of unlimited growth and has learned how to build order against the trend of disorder. The reversal of entropy, however, is destructive to the system unless the energy gained is used to produce other systems. The morality of the fifth stage is the "relinquishing of the power" but not of the products of this power. Young (1976b) explained, "There will come a time *in the lives of each of us* when we will go on or be destroyed, but this time will not come until we wield so much power that the misuse of it would destroy ourselves" (p. 216).

Most of us don't really know what happens at the sixth stage and beyond unless we have had these experiences of transcendence. We have some glimpse of the superhuman powers that exist by examining the events in the lives of those known to be evolved to higher levels: healings, appearances in different forms, and so on.

There is a corollary between my model of health as expanding consciousness and Young's conception of the evolution of human beings. We come into being from a state of potential consciousness, are bound in time, find our identity in space, and through movement we learn the "law" of the way things work and make choices that ultimately take us beyond space and time to a state of absolute consciousness.

Early in the development of my theory I was dealing primarily with the loss of freedom occurring in the 2nd, 3rd, and 4th substages of the process. Development of the physical self is necessarily binding in time and space. Movement provides a way of controlling one's environment. As physical disability brings about restriction in body movement, these losses of freedom become even more apparent. The restrictions in movement-space-time force an awareness that extends beyond the physical self. This awareness corresponds, I think, to the inward, self-generated reformation that Young speaks of as the turning point of the process. It comes about when the things that have worked for us in the past no longer work. We have to seek answers that are different from what we have previously considered "progress." The new awareness comes from a limitation of self that at the same time becomes a process of inner growth, a transformation. Land (Ainsworth-Land, 1982) pointed out that in transformation, *the old rules no longer apply.* One experiences the disconnectedness that is associated with pain (or disease or other forms of disruption). Things seem to be falling apart. This is the disorder, or disequilibrium, that is the necessary predecessor of a new order, or higher level of consciousness. There is a tendency to want to hold on to the old rules, but the need is to let go into a new realm. We need to be able to tolerate the uncertainty and ambiguity that precedes the clarity of the evolving pattern.

The next stage is the throwing off of centeredness, or concerns with one's own self, one's own boundaries, or space. It is recognition that one's essence extends beyond the physical boundaries and is in effect boundarylessness, as one moves to higher levels of consciousness. Transcendence, defined by Reed (1991) as expansion of self-boundaries and orientation to broadened life perspectives and purposes, is relevant here.

Progression to the 6th stage involves increasing freedom from time. This may be experienced in a sense of expanded time, a dilatation of a moment of time as we know it. Young (1976a) speculated that the reversal of time as we know it might be considered an inverse of time. If "normal" time (T) is long, then the inverse 1/T would be very short: eternity in an instant. He added that in a photon, energy is inversely proportional to time and implies that in an "anti" world, there might be unlimited energy in an instant of time. The experience of expanded time is one of going more deeply into the present and having the experience of all time.

The last stage is absolute consciousness, which has been equated with love. In this state all opposites are reconciled. This kind of love embraces all experience equally and unconditionally: pain as well as pleasure, failure as well as success, ugliness as well as beauty, disease as well as non-disease.

The process of learning the "law" (the new rules), reversing entropy and moving toward higher levels of consciousness may appear as quanta of action, each at higher levels of interaction.

Chapter Four

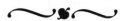

Manifestations of Expanding Consciousness

Research addressing the theory of health as expandang consciousness began with methods designed to describe and test
the relationships between selected major concepts: movement
and time in relation to consciousness (Newman, 1972; Newman, 1976; Newman, 1982; Newman & Gaudiano, 1984; Tompkins, 1980). The major concepts of the theory were abstracted
from the real world in which they were embedded and con-
verted into manipulable entities. I then tried to extrapolate the
results of such research into meaning related to the real world
situation. I sensed, even at the time this was happening, that
something was missing, but I forced myself to meet these external demands and was able to extract some meaning from
the research, particularly as it related to time as an index of
consciousness.

These methods were derived from a post-positivist approach and sought to meet the traditional scientific criteria of
objectivity and control. It took several iterations of this type of
research, including the work of others seeking to test this theoretical model (Engle, 1984; Engle, 1985; Mentzer & Schorr,

1986; Schorr, 1983; Schorr & Schroeder, 1991) to reveal the in-
congruency of these methods with the unitary-transformative
paradigm (Newman, Sime & Corcoran-Perry, 1991) that
guided the theory. When Engle followed my methods and
concluded that the faster one moves, the healthier one is, I
realized with sudden clarity that this conclusion reflected a
different paradigm than the one that I embraced (acknowledging now that I had not at that point been able to articulate the
paradigm in terms of method). The basic assumptions of my
theory centered on pattern: wholeness identified in pattern;
behavior as an indication of pattern; and expanding consciousness as seen in the evolving pattern (the process of
health). So, in the case of movement, it was not a dichot-
omized view of health as faster or slower movement; it was a
matter of identifying the *pattern* of movement and the *meaning*
of that pattern for the person.

The traditional scientific paradigm calls for predictable outcomes to situations, outcomes that have the potential to "fix"
problems. The new paradigm calls for action evolving out of
pattern recognition.

With that caveat, I will identify some examples of time,
space and movement, factors that relate to the deterministic
arm of Young's spectrum, and then attempt to elaborate the
transcendent phase by examples from more recent work on
patterning and pattern identification. The relevant task regarding the deterministic data is to see the concepts of movement-space-time in relation to each other, all at once, as
patterns of evolving consciousness. The varying dimensions
of movement-space-time portray configurations of consciousness evolving to higher levels.

TIME AND TIMING

The rhythm of living phenomena is a vivid portrayal of the embeddedness of matter (consciousness) in space-time. In 1965, Stephens challenged nursing to consider the relevance of temporal patterns in patient care. She described some of the rhythmic phenomena in human beings and animals and the possible hazards of drug and radiation therapy if the varying susceptibility of the organism during the 24-hour daily cycle is not taken into consideration. Data were available, for instance, on a drug that has a fatal effect at one point within the circadian cycle and a therapeutic effect at another point. She exhorted that more attention be given to the rhythms of people and the effects of the demands of the "therapeutic" regimen, particularly within an institutionalized environment. Now, almost 30 years later, there is little indication that consideration is given to the varying effectiveness of health care activities in relation to the client's cycles of receptivity.

Nowhere is the conflict of different time patterns more evident than in the bureaucratic system of the hospital. The timing of activities within a complex system such as a large hospital is indeed an intricate task and has become even more intense with the shortened hospital stays imposed by the cost-cutting strategies since 1983. Diagnostic and treatment activities, along with nursing care and food service, are woven into an intense program for each patient, geared to efficiency for the system, with little consideration of the temporal pattern of the person who is the recipient of these services.

The following example occurred in the days before these tight time restrictions were imposed on hospitals. Imagine what it would be like under today's restrictions.

A 19-year-old East Indian youth with a severe case of arthritis was considered "uncooperative" by the staff of an inpatient rehabilitation facility. He frequently refused to eat supper when it was served. He drank the tea on his tray and later ordered pizzas or similar foods to be brought in from restaurants. The next morning he would complain of gastrointestinal disturbances and, consequently, not be able to go to physical therapy. Investigation of the young man's usual pattern of activities revealed that he was accustomed to tea at 5:00 p.m. (hospital suppertime) and dinner around 8:00 (the time he would have meals brought in from outside). He was accustomed to highly seasoned food (like pizza) and did not like the relatively bland hospital fare. He preferred sedentary activities, such as reading, particularly in the morning hours (when he was scheduled for physical therapy), but if necessary, was willing to engage in physical activity in the afternoon. This young man was striving, probably inadvertently, to maintain his own life style and activity pattern, but in doing so incurred the wrath of the staff because their plans for his care were thwarted. In this situation nobody won: the staff could not accomplish their tasks and he was deprived of the rehabilitation services for which he was hospitalized. How different this situation could have been if his temporal patterns had been considered in his program of care.

Time is also a symbol of status. How much discretion people have in determining the way they spend their time is an indication of their status and power. When patients are made to wait for health care services, the message is clear as to who is important and who is not. Several years ago I met a man who found it impossible to coordinate his time pattern with that of the staff. He was quadriplegic and had been given a motorized wheelchair in an effort to mobilize him. Initially he was enthusiastic about the chair but later hardly ever got out of bed. The nurse viewed him as a complainer. The patient's view was that he was afraid to stay up for more than 3 to 4 hours because of the danger of pressure sores and he had difficulty getting assistance from the staff at the time he wanted to get up (and down). According to him, the staff preferred to get all the patients up early in the morning and then back to bed either early in the afternoon before the shift change or later in the afternoon when the next shift's staff could handle it. Neither of these times was congruent with his needs: He was not ready to get up until around 1:00 (too late, according to the morning shift workers) and was afraid that even if they got him up at that time, he might be left up too long before the evening staff were ready to help him back to bed. He did have frequent complaints of stomach pain, which got worse when he became upset over his situation. This patient's mobilization was blocked by his inability to articulate his time pattern with the task orientation of the staff. The increasing frustration he experienced was accompanied by increased stomach pain, and subsequently an increased need to stay in bed. He was caught in a vicious cycle, a Catch 22.

There is considerable evidence that people's temporal patterns are highly individualistic and have a bearing on their response to other people, their receptivity to therapy, their ability to learn new tasks, and their feelings about themselves. The above examples represent the power struggles patients and staff get caught in when the patients are attempting to express their own temporal patterns and the result impinges upon the staff's need to perform their work in a routine way.

More recently, timing is being recognized as a crucial factor in the effectiveness of nursing care, at least in long-term relationships in the home (Newman, Lamb & Michaels, 1992).

Freed from the usual bureaucratic time constraints, the nurse and client are able to orchestrate the timing of their interactions for optimal growth and change according to the client's needs and readiness. Here is what a nurse case manager had to say about it:

> When . . . [the client was] ready to express her feelings of confinement and explore options for opening her world, I made weekly home visits. When she returned to insulin use, I made weekly home visits plus three to four telephone calls per week for about one and a half months. During times when she let me know in her ways that it [was] not her time for change, I allowed the interval between visits to increase to a month and relied on her to call me if needed (Newman, Lamb & Michaels, 1992, p. 406).

Sensitivity to knowing when the need is there to connect with the client and when "This is enough," is an important skill for nurses to acquire.

After years of research on interactional synchrony, Condon (1980) made a strong case for individuals as *participants* in a complicated organization, a kind of web, of space-time: "The individuals do not create that order but participate in it. They 'live into' the forms and experiences which surround them and these forms become part of their very being" (p. 56). This description is consistent with the assertion that matter is a precipitate of the underlying pattern of consciousness, the implicate order.

INTEGRATION VIA MOVEMENT

Movement is a pivotal choice point in the evolution of human consciousness. Movement is the natural condition of life.

When movement ceases, it is an indication that life has gone out of the organism. The consciousness that characterizes any form of life is expressed in movement. It is through movement that the organism interacts with its environment and exercises control over its interactions. It is the fullest expression of consciousness in matter. Bohm (1981) regarded movement as the immediate experience of the implicate order: We do not know how we move, but when we wish to go somewhere, our imagination displays the activity. When we come into being in this physical world, we exist in time and space with a limited sense of self. Through movement we expand our knowledge of ourselves and others and the environment. When we reach the choice point when movement (both physical and social) is no longer an option, we learn to transcend the limitations of time-space-movement to higher levels of consciousness.

Kinesthetic consciousness is identical with the manifest dimensions of the world, a "world consciousness" (Mikunas, 1974, p. 11). In this sense, movement is not thought of as a succession of bodily locations but as a pattern of the total dance present in each movement, like a holographic view of the universe in which all of space-time is captured in any one place-movement. Every gesture is an indication of the silent dimension of the implicate order. The quality and rhythm of facial expression, body movements, and voice mirror our consciousness and the meaning we give reality (Gottlieb, 1982; Seagel, 1982).

The pattern of movement reflects the overall organization of thoughts and feelings of a person. Just as muscle activity is characterized by preparation-action-recovery, so an individual's overall pattern of movement reflects this inner organization and communicates the harmony of one's pattern with the environment (Hall & Cobey, 1974). The cycle of preparation-action-recovery becomes a spiral of development of our consciousness throughout the life span.

Rhythm is basic to movement:

> At the heart of each of us, whatever our imperfections, there exists a silent pulse of perfect rhythm, a complex of wave forms and resonances, which is absolutely individual and unique, and yet which connects us to everything in the universe. (Leonard, 1978, pp. xii)

Language reflects the rhythm of one's personal tempo, and this rhythm is reflective of both the rhythm of the person and the rhythm of the interpenetrating culture. When one cannot establish a mutually satisfying rhythm of relating, it is difficult if not impossible to communicate. When two people are relating well, the rhythm of the speaker is shared by the listener in a kind of mutual dance of empathy. The listener is not reacting or responding to the speaker but is *one with* the speaker. At the exact fraction of a second the speaker resumes talking, the listener begins his or her series of synchronized movements (Condon, 1980).

Hall (1984) reported a problem of blacks and whites in becoming synchronized with each other and attributed this difficulty to the feel or rhythm of the talk, not the words. The difference reported may have been a function of the shared (or lack thereof) rhythm of the culture. Leonard (1978), reporting Paul Byers' research, observed what appeared to be an angry shouting match between the chiefs of two villages in South America. The timing of the exchange, however, was very precise and revealed a synchronized talk dance. This synchronization has a biological effect of making the interactants feel good about what they're doing and about each other. Moving in synchrony with someone else, as in playing a musical instrument in an orchestra, singing in a choir, or marching in a parade, brings with it a feeling of closeness and unity with a greater whole.

The rhythm of movement is an integrating experience. When one's natural movement tempo is altered, as by trauma or by diseases of the neuromusculoskeletal system, one's perception of space-time also changes. My early research (Newman, 1972, 1976) was based on Piaget's thesis that time is a function of movement. When the participants walked at rates considerably slower than their natural walking rate, they felt that less time had passed than when walking at their natural rate. This relationship was supported by Tompkins' (1980) research, in which she simulated restricted movement by the application of knee and ankle braces. If this sense of altered time perception occurs in situations of natural variations in movement tempo, it implies the presence of conflicting rhythms among people of varying movement tempos.

Hall and Cobey (1974) described all body movement "in terms of that which is directed outward and that which is directed inward, in terms of attacking and defending, or more broadly, proceeding and yielding" (p. 6). This phenomenon was very apparent when, early in the development of specialized motorized wheelchairs, men who were long-time high-level quadriplegics regained some independent mobility. Before receiving these chairs, these men had been confined to manual wheelchairs and were dependent on others for their movement from place to place. When they became able to operate the chairs themselves, they experienced the freedom of visiting others when they wanted to, and more importantly, terminating the visit when it was no longer desirable to stay. Few of us stop to consider the control that movement affords us, to approach and withdraw as we please.

There are many situations in which this type of restriction of freedom occurs. The most obvious are those in which persons are incapacitated by chronic disease and are no longer able to pursue their previous activities. New parents are confronted suddenly with the loss of freedom entailed with their parenting responsibilities. Others, physically able but educationally or culturally deprived, find movement out of a circumscribed space-time difficult. Even though much progress has been made in readmitting the elderly to the mainstream of society, many senior citizens find certain avenues no longer open to them: their work, former companions, their family. These dimensions of their life space have become restricted.

My mother's incapacitation with amyotrophic lateral sclerosis made me very much aware of what restricted mobility means in terms of space and time. Not only was my mother not free to move about in space or to control her own time, but these restrictions applied also to me, the primary caregiver. The freedom to come and go as one pleases, when one pleases, is taken for granted until circumstances render that movement impossible or unwise. Restriction of movement forces one into a realm beyond space-time. The old ways of living and relating don't work anymore. One is confronted with one's own inner resources, the quality of one's relationships, and one's ability to live in the present. The developmental task is to learn the new rules as we are transformed beyond space-time in the movement to higher consciousness.

EXPANSION OF SPACE-TIME

Bentov's conceptualization of the relationship of subjective time to objective time (clock time) gave meaning to the findings of my studies of time perception as support for expanding consciousness across the life span (Newman, 1976, 1982). According to Bentov (1978), when an individual's subjective time is greater than objective time (say the *experience* of 4 seconds in 1 second of clock time), this ratio would indicate a higher level of consciousness than for someone whose subjective time equals clock time (1 to 1). The greater subjective time is experienced as a kind of dilatation or stretching of time, such as one experiences in a dream state. One has the experience of having a lot of time available in a short period of clock time. Athletes have reported this kind of experience, as is depicted in this account of a quarterback's feeling that he had all the time in the world to survey the field and target his pass:

> At times, I experience a kind of clarity that I've never seen described in any football story; sometimes time seems to slow way down, as if everyone were moving in slow motion. It seems as if I have all the time in the world to watch the receivers run their patterns, and yet I know the defensive line is coming at me just as fast as ever, and yet the whole thing seems like a movie or a dance in slow motion. It's beautiful. (Brodie, cited by Smith, 1975, p. 187)

The clarity that John Brodie felt illustrates the expanded consciousness associated with expanded time.

The basic element of reality is, according to Bohm (1980, p. 207) "a *moment* which, like the moment of consciousness, cannot be precisely related to measurements of space and time, but rather covers a somewhat vaguely defined region which is extended in space and has duration in time." Each moment has an explicate order and also enfolds all others, meaning that each moment of our lives contains all others of all time. Just as in the earlier illustration that elements separated in space are noncausally and nonlocally related, this introduces a new notion of time. Moments separated in time are also projections of a larger interconnected reality and may present themselves in varying orders of sequencing.

Our notions of causality rely on a linear, sequential view of time, our confidence in continuity, and do not encompass the basic tenets of evolution and quantum theory, that order and reason are based on a notion of randomness (Jones, 1982). Jones asserts: "but first the point (chaotic, unified, dimensionless, timeless experience) must become the interval. How? This is the fundamental act of creation, of the movement from unmanifest to manifest" (p. 97). The notion of causality depends on a particular view of space and time, motion in time through extended space. In a nondimensional totality-point, such as Jones suggests, no causal explanation can exist, since everything is everything else. Even the idea of relationship is no longer meaningful.

My early experiments relating movement to time perception were locked into a physical, linear view of movement-space-time. I rather quickly became dissatisfied with time estimation as a measure of the larger concept of time but could see it as some sort of indicator of the basic rhythm (pattern) of a person. The tentative findings, that subjective time increases with age, were contrary to prevailing theory based on a physiological mode. They required another explanation, a new paradigm, one that transcends the limitations of the linear, physical notions of space-time.

Schorr, too, found the quantitative, analytic approach used to test the theory of health as expanding consciousness inadequate to capture the nature of the theory and suggested that qualitative methods may be more appropriate (Schorr, Farnham & Erwin, 1991). She and her colleagues found a theme of hopefulness in elderly women in spite of the presence of chronic disease, diminished functional ability and decreased control over daily activities; they interpreted this configuration as evidence of transcendence of the physical self.

Friedman (1983) introduced an interesting view of space-time as an indicator of how one views oneself. His conceptualization went beyond the usual idea of self-concept and was presented as a measure of transpersonal development, or self-expansiveness. The self is seen as inextricably embedded in the universe. Friedman built on Deikman's view that the self is experienced in terms of the space-time of the world, in terms of all the things included in the zone of personal organization. The sense of identity is enlarged or contracted in terms of *extension beyond the here-and-now.*

I see these manifestations of space-time-movement as indicators of consciousness and offer the following examples. The women, from a semirural, middle-class setting, were asked by nurses to tell their stories of their lives. The interview data were subsequently analyzed in terms of the space-time-movement interactions:

1. Mrs. V. made repeated attempts to *move* away from her husband and to *move* into an educational program to become more independent. She felt she had no *space* for herself and she tried to distance herself (*space*) from her husband. She felt she had no *time* for leisure (self), was overworked, and was constantly meeting other people's needs. She was submissive to demands and criticism of her husband.

2. Mrs. K. has decreased her activities (*movement*) outside of home (work, church) and appears to be separating herself from others (building up *space* around herself). Her husband is away from home most of the time. She seems to be taking some form of sedatives or alcohol and sleeps most of the time (altering *time*).

3. Mrs. L is viewed as a "driving personality" (*movement*) and is very active but reluctant to *move* outside her own area. She cannot tolerate her husband or boss in "her *space*." She is very controlled in her use of *time*. She has no one with whom she can communicate openly.

4. Mrs. C. has very little activity outside the home (*movement, space*) except for her work. She has no private *space* ("cannot go to the bathroom alone") and no *time* alone. She has no social life and finds her interactions controlled by her husband and child.

These examples reflect a diminished sense of self as reflected in contracted, almost nonexistent space-time-movement, a reflection of the pattern of consciousness. The pattern of being controlled by others with little sense of one's own identity corresponds to the binding stage of Young's spectrum of the evolution of consciousness.

Survivors of murder victims undergo, according to Cowles (1988), intense personal transformation in terms of both physical world expansion (new, often disorganized environments) and personal expansion (intense emotional response to loss and search for meaning). These situations may be viewed as examples of the transformation that occurs when chance disruptive events propel the person into a disorganized, unpredictable fluctuation that provides the opportunity for creative restructuring (Prigogine, 1976). They also exemplify the relevance of extending the pattern focus beyond the individual. Often people ask how the theory of expanding consciousness can apply to catastrophic situations. The answer lies in broadening the focus beyond the individual to the meaning of their relationships with others.

THE CHOICE POINT AND BEYOND

The experience of life-threatening diseases and other disruptive events is associated with transcendence (Reed, 1991) and can be a turning point in the evolution of consciousness. LeShan (1989) saw cancer as a turning point in people's lives in experiencing themselves more fully. Self expansion was borne out in women who had been diagnosed with breast cancer (Moch, 1990). These women described ways in which they had become more sensitive to their own needs. They felt closer to others and were more receptive to others' expressions of caring. In general, they felt a greater connectedness and a greater appreciation of life. The enhanced quality of their interactions was seen as an indicator of the expansion of consciousness.

Other persons diagnosed with cancer told stories that illustrated their being caught in the bind of living their lives for others, unable to experience the essence of their own being (Newman, *unpublished*). In the crisis of cancer and the reality of their own mortality, several were able to open up to more meaningful relationships. Transcendence of the limitations of the disease does not necessarily mean freedom from the disease; it does mean more meaningful relationships and greater freedom in a spiritual sense. These factors are considered an expansion of consciousness.

Cunningham (1993), based on both his scientific background and his own encounter with cancer, has related his search for meaning in the experience of cancer. He pointed out the necessity of a new paradigm of interconnectedness of all that there is, one that goes beyond cause-effect. His work with cancer patients supports a life story approach to identify patterns of behavior and discover meaning, thereby learning to "sing one's own song."

Persons with coronary heart disease characteristically fit the Centering stage of Young's spectrum, one characterized by seeking power and position for oneself (Newman & Moch, 1991). Confrontation with the limitations of the disease and their own mortality became a turning point for some. Expansion of consciousness took place as they were able to let go of the striving for self, and seek to learn the rules of the new reality beyond space-time.

Men, confronted with a diagnosis of HIV/AIDS and experiencing other factors associated with the disease, found themselves at a turning point of reflecting upon the meaning of their lives and their relationships (Lamendola & Newman, 1994).

The movement from Binding to Centering to Choice Point and beyond seems to occur more readily for some than others. Persons whose entire lives have been bound in pleasing others and following the rules of a bureaucratic society find it more difficult to let go of the old rules and discover the new. But loving, caring help can facilitate the opening up of the heart to new possibilities.

BEYOND SPACE-TIME

Most of us can only speculate about the higher levels of consciousness portrayed in both Young's and Bentov's models.

According to Bentov (1978) it is possible to learn to interact with the whole spectrum of reality; there are meditative techniques that will facilitate movement into the astral realm. But Bentov warned that care must be taken not to go unprotected into this plane; an experienced teacher is required. Once emotional problems have been worked out, the evolution of human consciousness progresses to the mental level. At the mental level "the balanced mind" and the search for knowledge are dominant. The only emotion allowed is love.

Moss (1981) too equated expanded consciousness with deeper love. This kind of love:

> . . . is not something we can want . . . like we want a bicycle, or power, or even freedom from disease. This love belongs to the whole of self. . . . Those who approach naïvely or from an unconscious selfishness will turn back at the first experience of this love's tendency to bring forward the repressed and the lowly equally as it reveals the beautiful and the lofty. Much that we would never want to think within us will come forth in the light of these deeper forces. (p. 9)

> For the mature individual who is ready for this step, the art of living is the conscious loss of control, the letting go of the obsession with self, the surrender into being, the opening of the heart. (pp. 10–11)

The experience of real love involves extending our boundaries:

> What transpires then in the course of many years of loving (of extending our limits) . . . is a gradual but progressive enlargement of the self, an incorporation within of the world without, and a growth, a stretching and thinning of our ego boundaries. In this way the more and longer we extend ourselves, the more we love, the more blurred becomes the distinction between the self and the world. (Peck, 1976, p. 95)

This extension of oneself to incorporate and nurture another was illustrated in West's (1984) exploration of the experience of mothers of developmentally disabled children. Expecting to find these mothers harried by their responsibility and depressed by the limitations placed on them in the care of their children, she found instead that many of these mothers considered their experience as "special" and themselves as "chosen." They considered their experience as a "growing up" period in which they learned to be more mature, more giving and understanding, and more compassionate for other people. They felt that the presence of the child was a positive influence on the whole family and gave them purpose in life.

These mothers were able to embrace their present situation and allow themselves to be transformed by it. They were able to go beyond themselves and beyond reason into a new order of reality, a new level of consciousness. At this new level, defeat, failure and vulnerability are equally as important as success, power and gratifying relationships. Winning is not important; experiencing the moment fully is (Moss, 1981).

★ ★ ★

In the model of health as expanding consciousness it does not matter where one is in the spectrum. There is no basis for rejecting any experience as irrelevant. The important factor is to be fully present in the moment and know that whatever the experience, it is a manifestation of the process of evolving to higher consciousness.

Chapter Five

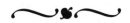

The Nature of Pattern

*P*attern is information that depicts the whole, understanding of the meaning of all the relationships at once. It is a fundamental attribute of all there is and reveals unity in diversity (Rogers, 1970).

An understanding of pattern is basic to an understanding of health. From the moment we are conceived to the moment we die, in spite of changes that accompany aging, we manifest a pattern that identifies us as a particular person: the genetic pattern that contains information that directs our becoming; the voice pattern that is recognizable across distances and over time; the movement pattern that identifies a person known to us a long way off even though no other features can be seen. These patterns are among the many explicate manifestations of the underlying pattern. It is the pattern of our lives that identifies us, not the substance that goes into making up that pattern. Ability to comprehend the unitary nature of human beings is enhanced as the concept of pattern is understood.

Pattern is relatedness and is self-organizing over time, i.e., it becomes more highly organized with more information. With increasing information, there is a more complex pattern of relationships. The pattern of relationships that characterized one's childhood, while enduring in some essential way, is different from the pattern at later stages of development. Each pattern is time specific *and* contains information which is enfolded from the past and which will unfold in the future.

Characteristics of patterning include movement, diversity, and rhythm. The pattern is in constant movement or change; the parts are diverse and are changing in relation to each other; and movement is rhythmic. The process of patterning occurs in the interpenetration of human energy fields as transformation takes place. The interference pattern of interacting waves forms a new pattern of the whole.

The ground, or background, of particular forms is equally as important as the form itself. We are able to recognize patterns by variations in contrast, e.g., the many subtleties of light and dark or of loud and soft. If the contrast is too slight or occurs over a long, extended period, we may not be sensitive to the pattern.

Gregory Bateson (1979), within the context of his concern about "the pattern which connects" (p. 12), was adamant that pattern cannot be understood by simple measures of quantity: "It is impossible, in principle, to explain any pattern by invoking a single quantity. But note that a *ratio between two quantities* is already the beginning of pattern" (p. 58). Bateson regarded the difference between number and quantity as profound. He regarded number as being in the same world of thought as pattern. The way to recognize number is to count, and counting is a form of pattern recognition and is discontinuous.

Quantity, on the other hand, is continuous and belongs in the world of analogic and probabilistic computation.

To illustrate that pattern and quantity are different logical types, Bateson suggested imagining an island with two mountains on it. When the ocean rises (a quantitative change), the island may become two islands. The qualitative pattern was latent before the quantity effected a change. When the change occurred, it was sudden and discontinuous. This example reminds me of situations in which the qualitative pattern of, say, a disease is latent, and then some quantitative change occurs, and the disease pattern manifests itself in a sudden and discontinuous event.

The whole of a person, or of a universe, is a pattern in which the parts cannot stand alone as separate. Entities, in and of themselves, provide only limited understanding. They are fictions of language, or of our mental models, for the purpose of figuring and describing. The important factor is the relationship between the entities. In music, for instance, the notes are incomplete without the rhythm of relationship between them. An adequate understanding of patterns cannot be reduced to an understanding of the properties of parts. What is primary is the self-regulating transformation by which the parts are continually being articulated in an everchanging whole. The changing pattern of a kaleidoscope may help to visualize this phenomenon.

PATTERN RECOGNITION

Pattern recognition comes from within the observer—which means that with any set of data or sequence of events, an infinite number of patterns are possible. If someone offers you the sequence of numbers—2,4,6,8—you will more than likely perceive a pattern of even numbers and predict that the next number will be 10. However, the pattern might be 2,4,6,8,11, 13,15,17,20,22,24,26 and so on. You are the one perceiving the pattern and the pattern will be changed by new information, or by anything that forces a new perception of it, like a change in context. For example, a behavior means one thing at age 5 and another at age 25. The nature of this phenomenon is such that the pattern cannot be predicted *with certainty* because the additional information has not happened yet (Bateson, 1979, p. 31).

Sometimes the pattern cannot be seen all at once. For example, Bohm, in describing the underlying pattern of the implicate order, suggested imagining a drop of ink placed in glycerine between two concentric cylinders. If the cylinders are rotated so that the particles of ink are distributed throughout the glycerine, becoming invisible, the pattern might be considered implicit (enfolded). The particles are there, nevertheless, and will reappear (become explicit—unfolded) when the cylinders are rotated in the opposite direction. Bohm elaborated: ". . . the particle is only an abstraction that is manifest to our senses. *What is* is always a totality of ensembles, all present together, in an orderly series of stages of enfoldment and unfoldment, which intermingle and interpenetrate each other in principle throughout the whole of space" (Bohm, 1980, p. 184). We need to remind ourselves that our manifest reality is a small portion of the total enfoldment of the pattern in time-space.

Extending the time frame helps to reveal the pattern. The field of chronobiology demonstrates the importance of viewing phenomena over time. A body temperature that might appear to be "abnormal" if recorded at only one time of the day may represent merely the peak of a normal cycle, or the turning point in the healing process. So it is with other phenomena that may appear to be disruptive at the time of their occurrence, but if viewed within an extended time frame, represent the reorganizing activity that precedes a higher level of organization.

Seeing the pattern is facilitated by distance from the system, as when one views a maze from above. This perspective eliminates the duality of separate objects, which, from a high-level view, are dispensable. That pattern, in turn, is embedded in another pattern. This latter point can be seen when one switches from viewing the pattern of a person to the pattern of person-family or further to the pattern of person-family-community, and so on.

Viewed from the perspective of the larger pattern, the activity of particular foci are understood in terms of the activity of the total system. Clusters of alliances change in relation to the tasks that need to be done. When one comprehends the whole, knowledge of the parts becomes meaningful. When one understands the configuration which is a triangle, for example, knowledge of two sides and an angle gives one knowledge of the whole.

The paradox is that the whole can be seen in the parts. A specific event can be viewed as an example of a class of events, and in this way the most specific patterns of a person may serve as prototypes of the general overall pattern of the person. There is generality in the specific. When an expert clinician monitors a pulse, she or he perceives much more about the person than merely the number of heartbeats per minute. In the same way a person's manner of walking communicates much more about his or her general well being and relationship to the world than simply the number of steps taken per minute or the amount of space transversed. This assumption, that the whole can be seen in the part, is basic to the process of nursing recognition of the whole. The important thing to keep in mind is the presence of the unitary pattern.

The inability to discern pattern, such as when the pattern is irregular or erratic, is important and may reveal a process of reorganization or a cue to search for the larger pattern in which it is enfolded. An observation may represent different meanings at different levels of organization. Considering that the explicate manifestation of reality is a limited view of the larger multidimensional reality, we need to be attuned to the fact that the pattern we glimpse is in the process of unfolding.

RELEVANT METHODS OF INQUIRY

A paradigm based on pattern requires a method of inquiry that will reveal pattern. The search for new alternatives in the methodology of knowledge development is apparent in nursing as well as in nearly every field of social science. Vaill (1984–85), in criticizing the traditional models of management, asserted that ". . . the American behavioral sciences don't amount to much as guides to action" (p. 40), that little if anything is done as a consequence of "knowledge." The problem with the old method of science, according to Vaill, is a "facts and methods" approach: "The facts and methods of modern behavioral science don't deal with the things that matter to more and more people in action roles today" (Vaill, 1984–85, p. 41).

The crux of action is *meaning* and precludes a paradigm of

reason that detaches the observer from the observed. In situations where decisions and action are required, the person involved finds himself/herself in a situation of not knowing exactly what one wants to achieve or what means there are to achieve it. Action involves extemporization and is not for those who enjoy the mechanistic, hypothetico-deductive logic of the old paradigm. The old paradigm is about the general case. The new paradigm of action and being is about specific persons in specific situations.

These concerns are particularly relevant to nursing situations, which require decisions and action within unique, unpredictable situations. Vaill (1984–85) suggested what he calls "process wisdom," or "being in the world with responsibility," as an alternative to the knowledge gained from the old paradigm. Process wisdom involves openness and relationality:

> . . . we are talking about personal expressiveness; about a dynamic, holistic phenomenon not easily or fruitfully broken into elements and lists of key factors; that the process of understanding such a phenomenon and the process of improving the effectiveness of those who practice it cannot be a matter of objectivist science. (p. 46)

It also involves the capacity to be fully conscious of one's involvement with other consciousnesses. And thirdly, it involves something beyond what you know materially, a knowledge that what you are doing is somehow right.

The apparent clash between an analytical, inferential approach and an immediate, direct understanding of the pattern of a person is not new. Allport (1961) recognized the dilemma in the early sixties and was adamant that the scientific approach is necessary but incomplete without perception of the individuality of patterning:

> Inference theorists tell us that the conditions for knowing any 'particular' are fulfilled only when its 'universal' or class membership is recognized. This . . . means in effect that we cannot know Peter or Paul unless we fit him into stock-sized clothes. It means that we can know Peter only insofar as we can code him. He is, let us say, a white Protestant, a college male, mesomorphic in build, who has a hundred scores on a hundred personality tests, and can be tagged with general conceptual labels, such as *cordial, ardent, intense, extroverted.* All these classes, so the inference theories tell us, constitute Peter. But do they? The unit that is Peter has disintegrated into a mere powder of concepts. The continuity of Peter has been broken into discontinuous and static categories. His life . . . is reduced to my conceptual furniture. There is no way of reconstructing the true mobility and pattern of Peter from this debris of concepts. (pp. 531–532)
>
> The role of inference is especially apparent when there is a hitch in the course of comprehension. When Peter puzzles me by his behavior, I am likely to ask, "Now what made him do that?" It was an act incompatible with my previous perception of pattern. I desire to repair the structure. I seek parallel conduct from the stores of my previous experience. But even while I try one analogy after another, and draw tentatively this inference and that, my interest is always channeled toward a patterned understanding of Peter as a single individual. (p. 546)

The solution to the dilemma, according to Allport, is to find a conciliatory approach by which we establish a method that provides both knowledge *about* people and an understanding *of* them. Search for such a method is of paramount importance as we move into the new paradigm.

Chapter Six

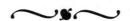

A Paradigm for Nursing Science

Despite a clear, consistent designation of holism as essential to the basic philosophical assumptions and practice realities of the discipline, the majority of research in nursing has been structured from positivist and post-positivist philosophical positions, which require analysis into parts (Newman, 1992a; Reynolds, 1988). A new paradigm based on movement of the undivided whole is needed to guide the development of nursing science. That paradigm was heralded by Rogers' science of unitary human beings.

When Rogers introduced her conceptual framework, which called for a distinctly different science—nursing science—based on assumptions of wholeness, pattern and unidirectionality, most nursing scientists could not envision such a science. The prevailing paradigm assumed that it was valid to analyze human beings into parts, reduce those elements to measurable entities, control and manipulate the parts, and try to extrapolate to the whole based on knowledge of the parts. Walker (1971) suggested that Rogers' call for wholeness was "asking for more than science [could] give," that is, asking for the experience of the phenomenon rather than a description.

Not even Walker knew then how relevant a forecast of the future of nursing science she had made.

Historically nursing has moved from addressing: (1) primarily the health of the body as affected by environmental factors to (2) the interaction of body-mind-environment factors in health, and more recently, to (3) health as an experience of the unitary human field dynamics embedded in a larger unitary field. These perspectives relate to different ontological positions. The first, stemming from the biophysical sciences, relates to a single paradigm, the positivist, objective view of science. The biopsychosocial approach involves multiple competing paradigms encompassing both objective and subjective phenomena, and falling primarily within the postpositivist perspective, which still holds to the control and predictability of the positivist view. The third perspective represents a radical shift and embraces a view of the human being as a unitary phenomenon unfolding in an undivided universe (Newman, 1992b).

THE UNITARY-TRANSFORMATIVE PARADIGM

This latter perspective has been identified as the unitary-transformative paradigm (Newman, Sime & Corcoran-Perry, 1991). From this perspective a phenomenon is identified by pattern and by interaction with the larger whole. Change is unidirectional and unpredictable as systems move through stages of organization and disorganization to more complex organization. Disruptive processes are viewed as a phase in the reorganization. Change is transformational, i.e., it involves the whole all at once, congruent with Parse's simultaneity perspective (Parse, 1987). Health is viewed as the evolving pattern of the whole, the explication of the unfolding implicate order.

Smith (1988) has provided a helpful analysis of the concept of wholeness. She pointed out that wholeness pervades most nursing conceptualizations, but from differing perspectives. The first perspective is wholeness as the sum of its parts and focuses on attributes of the person; the second focuses on the person as more than and different from the sum of the parts and focuses on identifying manifestations of the whole from the person's perspective of interrelationships with the environment. These perspectives, Smith argues, do not depict wholeness from a unitary perspective:

> The focus on attributes or experience does not take into account the person as inextricably tied to the environment in a dynamic web of interconnections. This view of wholeness is described as flowing motion. Person and environment are unitary; the person transforms with the environment and the environment transforms with the person. . . . one sees person with environment as a flowing, dynamic process with distinct recognizable features. Inquiry . . . focuses on the person-environment process as it is unfolding . . . [and] involves a creative leap to identify configurations of the rhythmical flow in the person-environment process as starting points for inquiry. (p. 94)

Nursing science sometimes has been referred to as human science. This designation admittedly emphasizes the human being as a whole rather than a sum or integration of parts, but may serve to separate the human being from the flow within the larger dynamic context. It is important to see the human being as unitary *and* as continuous with the undivided wholeness of the universe (Bohm's holomovement). There are no boundaries. This viewpoint is also important in visualizing the practicing nurse's participation as integral to the evolving pattern of the whole.

Bohm (1980) repeatedly emphasized the inseparability of the process of thought and the content of thought. There are certain fundamental changes in the way we think about things brought about by quantum theory:

> A centrally relevant change in descriptive order required in quantum theory is thus the dropping of the notion of analysis of the world into relatively autonomous parts, separately existent but in interaction. Rather, the primary emphasis is now on *undivided wholeness*, in which the observing instrument is not separable from what is observed. (p. 134)

The paradigm guiding nursing research and practice needs to be consistent with this new world order. The phenomena of our research and practice cannot be viewed in an action-reaction mode (Condon, 1980; Davis, 1982). They are co-acting, moving in shared rhythms, and we must learn to look at the interactive rhythm, something that cannot be seen when observing one person at a time. Butrin (1992) found it necessary to look at the experience of mutuality in nurse-client relationships in order to learn whether or not nurses of one culture could be effective with clients of another culture. It was not enough to set up in advance certain criteria of effectiveness as outcome measures pertaining to the client. It was necessary to attend to the experiences of both the client and the nurse in relation to each other in order to identify which experiences were congruent, which were incongruent, which were satisfying, and which were unsatisfying. The relationship was paramount—the connection between the two. Likewise Schmitt (1991) initially sought to interview the caregiver in elderly couples regarding the experience of giving and receiving support but quickly recognized the importance of participating with both members of the dyad in a mutually interactive fashion.

We are beginning to let go of the false dichotomy of investigator and subject, nurse and client, and are engaging in investigations in which the participants are our partners in revealing the evolving pattern. It makes sense that if we value self-determination and active participation in practice, then those conditions characterize our research. The most authentic encounter one has with another person is when that person is encountering oneself. Heron (1981), referring to his paradigm of cooperative inquiry, stressed the primacy of interpenetrating attention for the development of valid social knowledge. In an interactive, dialectical process, there can be no subject-object split: The concept of "objective" is obsolete, but so also is the concept of "subjective." Validity is a function of the relationship of the two (or more) persons: it is "we" knowledge.

DEVELOPING A METHOD CONSISTENT WITH THE PARADIGM

Previous attempts to identify pattern by analyzing clients' responses to questions in relation to the major concepts of the theory (movement, space, time) were successful in depicting the pattern of the whole in the sense of Smith's second perspective of wholeness, namely interaction of the person(s) with the environment, but failed to bring forth data that were meaningful in terms of the dynamics of the unfolding pattern and the nurse-investigator's participation in it. I realized, with the help of Susan Moch, that what we needed to solicit from individuals was what was most meaningful in their lives. After all, meaning is pattern. As the participants began to tell their stories of the people and events in their lives that were most meaningful to them, the dynamics of the pattern became apparent, both in terms of the unfolding nature of expanding consciousness and also in terms of the action potential of the moment. Bramwell (1984) employed a similar approach by obtaining life histories as a method of pattern identification and a process of intervention within a framework of health as expanding consciousness.

The need to capture a picture of the pattern of the *whole* of the person in interaction with the environment became a priority in the early work of the theory task force of the North American Nursing Diagnosis Association (NANDA) (Newman, 1984). As I worked with this way of seeing the whole, I realized that the pattern was evolving ver time and therefore could not be portrayed as one pattern ᴸ ᵗt, at the least, must be shown as sequential patterns over timᴇ (Newman, 1986b). In a pilot study intended to identify a methodology of pattern identification, Jim Vail, Richard Cowling, and I incorporated a diagram of sequential patterns over time as a way of organizing the data from the interviews regarding the meaningful events in the participants' lives (Newman, 1987b). We were able to portray the meaningful relationships in configurations at particularly important times in the person's life and to openly share this portrayal with the interviewee for confirmation, clarification, and revision.

The immediate experience of both the participants and the investigators came as a surprise. The persons being interviewed were quite expressive of the insight they experienced in reviewing their life pattern in this way. Participants in Bramwell's study, too, were able to obtain a global perspective of themselves, a process which led to integration, heightened self-awareness, and further creativity. An even greater revelation for us was the discovery that the interactive process engaged in with the client was transformative not only for the interviewee but also for us as the interviewers! (Obviously we had not fully relinquished the old idea of investigator-subject split until this experience.)

Our activities up to this point took place without any particular attention to theory. We simply asked the participants to tell their stories in a non-directive way. We organized the data chronologically and tried to portray the nature of the relationships in diagrammatic form just as they were described (e.g., loving, close, hostile, distant, and so on), without interpretation, but at the same time, noting any contradictions, similarities, or other relational qualities within the data.

After the evolving pattern had been identified and affirmed by the interviewee, we were free to examine it in regard to the theory of expanding consciousness. The quality of the relationships over time could be evaluated in terms of consciousness, defined as the quality and diversity of relationships with the environment.

This hermeneutic, dialectic approach (Guba & Lincoln, 1989; Moustakas, 1990) is consistent with the unitary-transformative paradigm. The method is dialectic and the nature of data being collected is dialectic. It seeks to capture the evolving, transformative nature of the nurse-client relationship. The *a priori* nature of theory in this praxis research is evident in that the researcher embodies the theory of expanding consciousness. By virtue of the interpenetrating field of nurse researcher and client, the theory is active in the dialectic.

Participants are encouraged to tell their stories in their own way and investigators are free to be authentic in response to them. Organization of the data in chronological order as a narrative (see Polkinghorne, 1988) is helpful in identifying the evolving patterns of people's lives and of the unfolding process. The data is interpreted from the *a priori* theoretical perspective of health as expanding consciousness.

The method is as dynamic as the paradigm. Included in the appendix is the protocol being used at the present time. It assumes a unitary, transformative nature as the reality of the process: two or more unitary beings engaged in the evolving patterning of their interconnected fields. The specific question(s) asked vary according to the focus of the study. The important point is that mutuality be established and that interviewees tell their stories as fully as possible. It is essential that the interviewer be fully present with an intent to know (to care) and to come from the center of her/his truth.

THEORETICAL PRESENTATION

How are we to interpret and communicate these data? Heron's call for presentational construing of the data is consistent with the focus on sequential patterns over time. Heron asserted that presentational construing includes and transcends propositional construing. Presentational construing portrays a sequence of presentations as a total process, as in listening to music or seeing the flight of a bird (Heron, 1981). It is a spatiotemporal whole that transcends the immediate space and time and is reminiscent of Bohm's description of the implicate order.

Heron did not dismiss a propositional approach as irrelevant:

> Too much propositional construing blinds researchers to the gestures of being. Too much presentational construing keeps

the archives of propositional knowledge empty . . . (p. 31) . . .
true propositions are asserted by those who know how properly to symbolize in words *shared experiences* of shared value . . .
(p. 12) (Emphasis added.)

The portrayal of sequential patterns over time for individuals
and their significant others is an example of presentational
construing. The pattern synthesized from many such patterns
of persons selected as having a common experience may provide the basis for propositions of shared experience.

Every time I start breaking things down into parts for the
sake of theory development, I realize that I lose something,
but nevertheless I will risk trying to illustrate the way I think
this process works. In a study of life patterns of persons with
coronary heart disease (Newman & Moch, 1991), each participant's pattern-of-the-whole was identified in terms of sequential patterns over time. These patterns could be considered
presentational construing; they also formed the basis for action emerging out of the recognition of the individual's evolving pattern. A synthesis of the life patterns within the group
revealed a common pattern of relationships. These latter relationships might be considered propositional construing, a
more general kind of archival knowledge.

To illustrate further, examples of presentational construing
can be seen in the sequential patterning of selected participants, all of whom were in a rehabilitation program following
myocardial infarction and/or coronary artery bypass surgery:

Carol,[1] a 59-year-old married woman with three adult children, recalled a lonely childhood when both her parents were
employed outside the home. She was responsible for many

---

[1]All client names in this section are pseudonyms.

household tasks, but felt she could never please her mother, who was very critical of what she did (Pattern$_1$ (P_1)). She married early and became totally ensconced in her role as wife and mother (of two daughters, one son) as dictated by the tenets of her church (P_2). She became estranged from her adult children when their life styles violated her religious beliefs and teachings, and this situation in turn brought about a block between her husband and her (P_3). Carol had a myocardial infarction a year ago, followed by coronary artery bypass surgery with post-operative complications. When asked what was most meaningful in her life, she answered, "My husband and my family," but quickly moved on to talk about herself and what she perceived to be her lack of accomplishment in her lifetime. She saw herself as having always been limited by her obligations to her family. She felt she had "missed the boat" regarding her own personal development and had never accomplished anything for herself. She felt she had failed because her children had rejected her teachings. She was unable to communicate her true feelings to her children. She saw herself as going round in circles like "a squirrel in a cage" (P_4).

When viewed from the theory of expanding consciousness, this woman was caught in the Binding Stage of Young's spectrum, literally going round in circles trying to meet the external expectations of the church and trying unsuccessfully to control the behavior of her children and her husband. The action potential for her is to let go of trying to meet those external demands (rules) and discover the new rules from within her own reality (identity).

Another participant, Allen, a 57-year-old man in his second marriage, exemplified the Centering Stage. This man was the last of seven children and talked about being worried at times that he would not have enough to eat (P_1). As he grew up, he worked hard to please his father and eventually took over the family business. He was also very active in volunteer work and became a "pillar" of the community. The most important thing to him was to be intensely involved in things, get them done "right," and be "first" in everything he did. He expressed pride in being in the center and at the helm of helping activities (P_2). Following his myocardial infarction he was faced with acknowledging that his strivings no longer worked, but he was still seeking to be No. 1 in other activities such as grandparenting (P_3). The need is to let go of the striving to be the center of activity, so that he can see beyond himself as the center and thus transcend his physical limitations.

A final example is Bob, a 39-year-old divorced man, who was feeling particularly successful at the time of his heart attack. He had been pretty much a loner as a child and adolescent, not close to his parents or to anyone else (P_1). He excelled in sports and in music, which was his primary love and to which he committed himself as a career. He did marry at age 25 but let his wife "slip away" because of his primary allegiance to his career (P_2). He experienced all of the same strivings for top position and perfection in sports and career, but when the heart attack occurred, he experienced the disruption as a Choice Point of meaning in his life and was transformed by the experience (P_3).

The purpose of the presentations of the evolving pattern of each of the participants' lives is to help them to gain insight into their pattern and reveal the action potential of the pattern.

The proposition from this data, as I see it, is drawn from the general themes that emerged: the need to excel, the need to please others, and the feeling of being alone. Stated specifically: Experiences associated with coronary heart disease are the need to excel, the need to please others, and the feeling of being alone. The propositional statement does not differ from that associated with the traditional scientific paradigms. When viewed from the standpoint of Young's spectrum of the evolution of consciousness, it groups the data and places it primarily at the Centering Stage of development. In contrast, the individual experiences may range from the Binding Stage to the Choice Point and beyond. The presentational constructions, therefore, provide the specificity of knowledge needed for practice, namely, a person's recognition of his/her specific pattern and the concomitant release, letting go, of the "old ways" that contract their being and inhibit movement in the new reality.

RESEARCH AS PRAXIS

I have concluded that nursing research must focus on the reality of practice. Research that produces data as outcome is not enough. Nursing research helps participants understand and act on their particular situations. The research portrays the emancipatory process of pattern recognition. This is research as praxis, defined as "thoughtful reflection and action that occur in synchrony, in the direction of transforming the world" (Wheeler & Chinn, 1984, p. 2). Recognition of pattern is essential to the process of expanding consciousness and is the key to nurses' being able to engage in this process with clients needing help.

The process of nursing practice is the content of nursing research. What we need to understand is the process of transformation from one point to another. In relation to my theory, the question is: what is the process of expanding consciousness? Sometimes it is difficult to see the pattern as expanding consciousness in the present moment. But even when the pattern appears to be disorganized or blocked, the eventual unfolding will come about as action at a higher level of consciousness.

We need to get beyond the idea that knowledge is somehow *foundational*, or like *building blocks*. Morgan (1983) equates the quest for knowledge with human practice:

> . . . when we engage in research action, thought, and interpretation, we are not simply involved in instrumental processes geared to the acquisition of knowledge but in *processes through which we actually make and remake ourselves as human beings*. (p. 373) (Emphasis added.)

Research as praxis captures the essence of the work that my colleagues and I have done in a search for pattern identification. It involves *a priori* theory:

> For praxis to be possible, not only must theory illuminate the lived experience . . . ; it must also be illuminated by their (the researched) struggles. Theory adequate to the task of changing the world must be open-ended, nondogmatic, informing, and grounded in the circumstances of everyday life; . . . (Lather, 1986, p. 262)

The necessity of *a priori* theory renders a strictly interpretive, phenomenological approach inadequate. There is an interpenetration between the researcher's embodied theory and the researched's understanding.

Chapter Seven

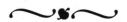

Practice: Order Out of Chaos

When health is conceptualized as the expansion of consciousness in a universe of undivided wholeness, intervention aimed at producing a particular result becomes a problem. To intervene with a particular solution in mind is to say we know what form the pattern of expanding consciousness will take, and we don't. Moss (1981), who declares himself a *former* general practitioner of medicine, asks where is the world going anyway, except round in circles. Somehow this bigger picture makes it easier to relax and enjoy an authentic involvement/evolvement with another person.

The usual concept of intervention is derived from the instrumental paradigm of medical science. It requires that the professional identify what is wrong with a client, why it is wrong, and then take steps to remedy the problem.

Nursing intervention is derived from a relational paradigm that directs the professional to enter into a *partnership* with the client, often at a time of chaos, with the mutual goal of participating in an authentic relationship, trusting that in the process of its unfolding, both will emerge at a higher level of consciousness. Reconsider the fluctuating pattern of dissipa-

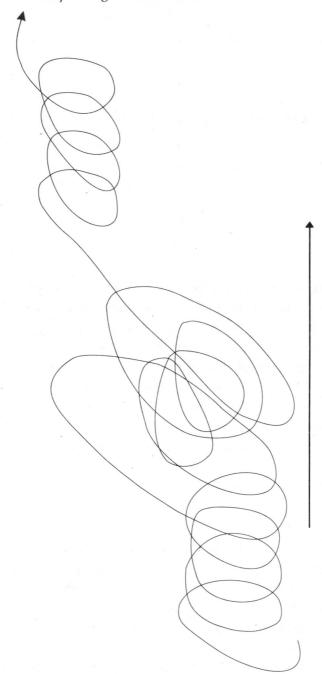

Period of nurse-client relationship from beginning of chaotic phase to stabilization at new level.

Figure 7.1   Nursing partnership with client during period of uncertainty and reorganizing.

tive structures (described in Chapter 3) with the nurse-client relationship extending through the period of chaos until order can be established (see Figure 7.1). People need a partner in this process.

The thing that brings people to the attention of a nurse is a situation that they do not know how to handle. They are at a choice point. Each of us at some time in our lives is brought to a point when the "old rules" do not work anymore, when what we have considered progress does not work anymore. We have done everything "right" but things still do not work. We come to a point when the old rules do not work and the task of life, *the crux of life*, is to learn the new rules (Bateson, 1979; Young, 1976). This means learning how to transcend a situation that seems impossible, to find a new way of relating to things, and to discover the freedom that comes with transcending the old limitations. The necessity of "hanging in there" in the midst of the uncertainty and ambiguity of the chaotic situation is an important factor in the healing process. One cannot regard the organized part as okay and the disorganized part as not okay. They are both part of the same process of expanding consciousness. We as nurses enter into the process with a client to be present with it, attend to it and live it, even if it appears in the form of disharmony, catastrophe, or disease.

The story of a young divorced woman (Marchione, 1986; Newman, 1987b) exemplifies how the health patterning and partnership with a nurse reflect the process of expanding consciousness. This woman, whom I will refer to as Kay, was solely responsible for the care of her two children and supported herself by providing day care for an infant and three other children. The incident that brought Kay to the attention of a nurse was the sudden death of the infant while being cared for by Kay. Shortly after the infant's death, a nurse contacted Kay and offered information about Sudden Infant Death Syndrome (SIDS). Kay asked for help in relating to her two children, aged two and five, who had witnessed the event and had become difficult for Kay to deal with. When the nurse visited the home, she found it in complete disarray, with the children fighting each other and their mother. Kay was tearful, felt fatigued, and wanted to be alone. She had lost interest in her children and was suffering from insomnia. The nurse offered some suggestions for immediate action regarding the children and invited Kay to attend a support group, which she later attended, and from which she received considerable comfort and support.

The nurse maintained periodic contact with Kay, and fifteen weeks later, although still sad about the experience of the infant's death, Kay had begun to reach out to others in her family and in the community.

Prior to the SIDS incident, Kay was feeling bored with her life. She was relatively isolated from adult interaction, having limited contact with her ex-husband and her family of origin, even though her mother and brother lived in the same vicinity (P_1). At the point at which the nurse entered the situation, Kay's pattern of interaction was one of disorganization, feelings of sadness, and guilt and frustration with her child care responsibilities (P_2). Through this experience she was able for the first time to reach out for assistance to her mother-in-law. She established a friendship with the parents of the infant who died. She learned to allow the children to discuss the experience of the infant's death and to ask questions freely. She felt as though she had become more outgoing and caring in her relationships with other people (P_3).

The evolving pattern of this period of Kay's life moves from a repetitive pattern of a relatively closed, low energy system to one of disorganization following the disruptive event of the infant's death, to a pattern of restabilizing at a higher level of functioning. The nurse participated in the patterning following the disruptive event and maintained contact with Kay until she was able to establish other mutually supportive relationships. When the nurse was asked what she thought she had done in the situation, she said she felt that she provided an organizing force. This sequential pattern corresponds to the process of dissipative structures: first the repetitive, predictable cycles, then the reorganizing phase precipitated by a chance disruptive event, and then stabilization at a higher level of functioning (see Figure 7.2). The process is ongoing.

The emphasis of other theorists' work can be seen in this situation: A transitional event, which Meleis (1993) views as central to nursing's concern; a period of uncertainty, during which the client has an opportunity to reorganize in a more meaningful way (Mishel, 1990); and the nurse as "a little point of light" within the confusion and vulnerability of illness or other disruptive event (Watson, 1987). The nurse was able to provide the information and support that Kay needed during the tumultuous period, from which Kay emerged at a higher level of interaction.

GIVING UP A PRESCRIBED AGENDA

The task for us as health professionals is to stop trying to change the world in accordance with our own image of what is healthy and instead "fall toward the center of ourselves" (Moss, 1981, p. 39). We need to give up the old agenda to fix things. The necessity for doing leads us into a pattern of con-

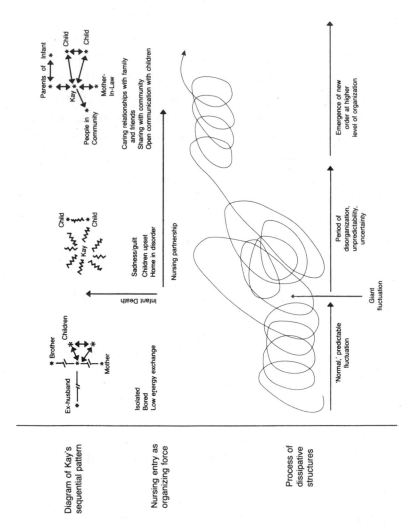

Figure 7.2 Relationship of Prigogine's theory to nursing intervention in evolving pattern of a selected client.

traction and diminished sensitivity. As one is able to let go of the old, restricted view of health and open up to the full spectrum of the whole, one's practice expands. One nurse case manager related:

> It was a personal and professional stretch to look at the whole . . . I'm sharing my experience with the person [client], [just] as what they're going through is offered to me. I hear things and recognize things in people that I wouldn't have before . . . (Newman, Lamb & Michaels, 1992).

Lamendola struggled with his role while conducting interviews as part of praxis research within this paradigm:

> I soon realized that all I had to do was "be there" and listen . . . I needed to let go of thinking I had to lead the interview in a direction or make the pain better or fix a problem. The purpose . . . was to allow a sense of the whole to emerge . . . (Lamendola & Newman, 1994).

He later contrasted this approach with what he had previously considered the fixed agendas of his practice role. The joy of nursing lies in being fully present with clients in the disorganization and uncertainty of their lives—an unconditional acceptance of the unpredictable, paradoxical nature of life.

It is impossible to know what a "successful" outcome will be other than that it is a shift from a concentration on self to a broader perspective that extends beyond self, a kind of universal perspective. It will be manifest in congruence between inner and outer experience and a greater capacity for love and relatedness in the world. The health professional's awareness of being, rather than doing, is the primary mechanism of helping: ". . . being with another person, willing to participate empathically in his/her experience, without becoming identified with it and without imposing any agenda, preconceived goals, or outcomes on the process" (Vaughan, 1979, p. 28).

Doberneck, a nursing clinician, related her experience of giving up her own agenda and being with clients, not to change anything but simply to be with them as they identified their concerns and the actions they wanted to pursue. She pointed out that things came up that were more central to their lives than what she might have had on her agenda. She admitted that she had to guard against a "doing" approach. It was not that she didn't do anything. In the process of her interaction with clients, she shared information regarding topics of concern to them, referred one patient to a physician on the basis of symptoms of heart disease, discussed one patient's concerns regarding the anticipated death of her spouse, and helped a grandmother deal with a developmental crisis of her young adult grandson. Doberneck observed that if she could maintain an unconditional caring relationship long enough, a shift occurred when trust had been established. The relationship then felt somehow *lighter* and the distancing that had been characteristic of the relationship seemed to disappear.

HOLOGRAPHIC MODEL

A holographic model of intervention is consistent with the new paradigm. To comprehend this model it is helpful to review some of the basic elements of a hologram. A hologram contains an image in which the whole is written into each part; a three-dimensional image is produced by wavefront reconstruction. Light waves bouncing off an object interact with a pure light reference beam, and the resulting interference pattern is imprinted on the film. When another reference beam is projected through the film, the image of the object is recreated by the interference pattern of the film. This process is often explained by imagining the emanating waves that appear when two pebbles are thrown into water. As the waves radiate toward each other, they meet and interact and an interference pattern evolves. The interference pattern spreads and is a part of the whole of each of the previous patterns.

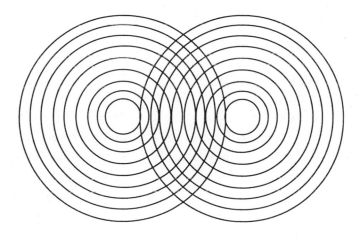

Figure 7.3 Interference pattern of waves emanating from two pebbles thrown in a body of water.

Now substitute two people for the two pebbles and imagine *the waves radiating from each person interacting with the other pattern and becoming an interference pattern that is part of each person's pattern:*

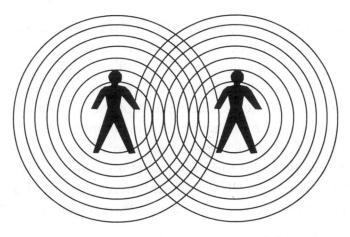

Figure 7.4 Interaction pattern of two persons: A holographic model of intervention.

The interference pattern continues and encompasses the whole environment. To be in touch with the other person and the environment, the task is to be *in touch with oneself, to sense into one's own pattern*. The observer and the observed are interpenetrating aspects of one whole. In a holographic view of the world the totality of existence is enfolded in each region of space-time. The order that has been recorded in the complex movement of electromagnetic fields (light waves) is present everywhere and enfolds the entire information of the universe in each region of space and time (Bohm, 1980).

The more we can sense into ourselves, to trust the information that is there, the clearer we will be in expressing our own truth and in knowing other persons. The thesis of this book is that the highest form of knowing is loving, and so we are admonished to love ourselves, a dictum not unfamiliar in spiritual teachings. Keen (1978) has commented on the partnership of science and religion in supporting the notion that each person is a microcosm of the macrocosm, with the implication: "Consider the enormity of the self each of us is invited to inhabit and love" (p. 88).

In a hologram, even though every part contains information about the whole, the smaller the part, the fuzzier the picture. The fuzziness of the pattern is sometimes experienced in the beginning of an interaction with another person when there is a sense of pattern or meaning that is not entirely clear. But the felt meaning will become clearer as one stays with the interaction and waits for the pattern to emerge.

In the medical paradigm, practice is divided into discrete parts: assessment, diagnosis, intervention; the emphasis is on the individual, either alone or in the context of family and environment. In the nursing paradigm there are no separate parts; the process is one of sensing in to the pattern of the whole. There is no permanent pattern of fixed form but a continuous flow of movements and relationships that merge into each other. Music gives us this sense of the moving, interpenetration of many rhythms and relationships. There are no separate parts; the individual field is continuous with the family and the environment.

PATTERN RECOGNITION

Pattern recognition occurs, as the holographic model suggests, by going into ourselves and getting in touch with our own pattern and through it in touch with the pattern of the person or persons with whom we are interacting.

Gendlin's (1978) process of focusing was a helpful starting point for me, but can be relinquished once one begins to trust the information always present in one's being. The process of focusing involves directed concentration on oneself, more specifically on the feelings one is aware of in the body. It may be a heaviness in the heart or stomach area, a pain in the shoulders or lower back, or something far more diffuse. The task is to concentrate on the feeling, to get in touch with it, and to try to explicate it by naming it. If the first name you give it does not feel right, you stay with it and continue to name it until your identification of the feeling coincides with the deeper non-verbal message of your body. When this congruence is reached, there is usually a total relaxing shift that occurs in your body, similar to that experienced when you finally remember something that you have been blocking on. The process of focusing and relaxing releases energy for growth even when you are not aware of what growth is occurring. The process may take a while and seem to be going nowhere, but if you can be patient and trust in the unseen, evolving pattern, it will emerge. If you are facilitating the process with someone else, you are acting like the reference beam in the hologram, making it possible for the interference pattern to occur and for pattern recognition to emerge.

The pattern may present itself as visual. Once while listening to a woman with cancer describing her experience of pain and fear while telling members of her family that she had received a diagnosis of cancer, I had a visual picture of her as the "sink" into which all of the fear of her family was flowing. From her description of previous interactions with her family, I sensed that this pattern of interaction was true for other situations. Previously she had been the strong member who could absorb the fear, but in this situation she was vulnerable and was pained by the contradiction between her own truth—a feeling of oneness and strength in the confrontation with the disease—and the fear she was sensing from her family. When

I related my "observation" of the sink to her, it felt right to her. Her bodily sensation was signaling the conflict inherent in the pattern, and she was relieved by this recognition and her ability to let go of the need to absorb the family's fear.

The nurse must be fully present with the client and wait for insight into the meaning of the pattern. To do this, one has to be committed to "standing in the center of one's truth" (Arguelles, 1987), i.e., being able to sense and communicate whatever is true for oneself in the moment. The question that has echoed over the years is, "But what does the nurse *do* in relation to the pattern?" The action indicated will become apparent only as the pattern becomes apparent. The action emerges from the "truth" discovered as clients find the center of their truth and discover the new rules that apply to their situations. Then *they* will know what to *do*. Smith (in press) related the tendency of African American families in a rural community to resist interactions emphasizing the need to "fix" things, since they did not identify their situations as "problems" affecting their health. "Staying healthy" for these families centered on finding meaning in life experiences, "an inner feeling of knowing what to do" (Smith, in press). When the insight occurs, no matter how complex the situation, the solution is simple. Litchfield (1993) interpreted action on the part of clients as evidence that pattern recognition had occurred. The action concomitant with the insight of pattern recognition was the transformative moment.

THE RHYTHM OF RELATING

Rhythm is a basic characteristic of pattern and a powerful factor in interpersonal relations. Pelletier (1978), recognizing the importance of timing in client relationships, drew an analogy of twirling balls on the end of a string. The point at which a ball is released determines the direction it will take. Being able to wait until the client is ready to move may be difficult; allowing the client to move in his or her own direction, which may be in conflict with the nurse's values or beliefs, may be even more difficult.

The rhythm of talking is an important consideration in interpersonal relations. The pauses in talking may be more relevant than the words. One encounter group technique involves persons forming two concentric circles, with the inner circle facing out and the outer circle facing in. Instructions are to face a partner and say "Hello," to which the partner responds with "Hello." This exchange is repeated several times until participants are instructed to move on to the next person in the circle, and the greetings are again exchanged. This simple experiment is very revealing in that after you have gone full circle, perhaps more than once, you have a good idea of which persons you are comfortable with and which ones jar your rhythm.

The person who interrupts a meaningful pause may be squelching an important idea or may never hear an important message that was forthcoming. We often think of the beats of the music or the utterances of a voice as the structure of the rhythm, but the nature of the pauses, or the silences between, are equally germane. Watson (1976) reinforces the importance of the silence between utterances in the lesson he learned from the djuru, an Indonesian native who was able to listen underwater to locate fish and predict tidal waves. The djuru instructed Watson to put his head underwater and listen. Watson relates the conversation:

"What did you hear?"
"Nothing."
"That was my trouble too."
"What?"
"I could not hear it."
"Hear what?"
"Nothing."

Watson continues:

> I could not teach myself to listen to the silence. The djuru can do this. He is trained to listen intently to nothing, because the secrets lie in the spaces between the sounds. He is able to listen when all is quiet and to look when there is nothing to see.
>
> I remembered . . . my insistence on being told exactly what each of the fish sounded like. He had made up metaphors to keep me happy, and they had. But now I felt rather ashamed. [He] watched my awareness grow, and he nodded sympathetically. A kingfisher swept by overhead, cutting across the lagoon with deep, irregular wingbeats, and it was only in the brief pause between each flurry of feathers and the next that I could be sure of the cool cerulean blue of its back.
>
> Long after it disappeared into the mangroves, I could still hear its loud rattling cry. It is a very distinctive sound which fills my head with the message "Kingfisher calling." But it was only in the silent moment between one proclamation and the next that I had time to think about the bird. It was only in the pauses that I was able to reflect on the relationship between the bird and me. (pp. 196–197)

The importance of attending to the silence between signals is crucial to getting in tune with one's inner voice, the pattern of oneself, one's consciousness. Watson's description of the djuru is a vivid portrayal of how one can become receptive to the larger pattern:

> There is no known sense organ that can give a man [sic] under-water the capacity for locating things precisely in the dark, or for responding appropriately to the precursors of a seismic wave. I believe he [the djuru] was able to do these things because he turned his whole body on and tuned in completely to the entire spectrum of information. He listened to the waves and heard not only their news but signals in the silence between them. He measured the intervals and established a beat produced by interference between these waves and others elsewhere. And in this way he put his consciousness in a position to transcend the physical limits of information transfer. (p. 199)

THE NURSE-CLIENT RELATIONSHIP

The nurse-client relationship is a rhythmic coming together and moving apart of the client and the nurse (Martin, 1985). The process occurs in three steps: (1) meeting, (2) forming shared consciousness (the interpenetration of the two fields), and (3) moving apart. The meeting occurs when there is a mutual attraction of the nurse and client via congruent patterns. The forming of shared consciousness is a sharing of the whole of each person to form a connection, the feeling of "clicking" with another person, or being "in synch." Martin points out that the nurse needs to be fully present: "100 percent observer and 100 percent participant," for the meeting "to gel" and "form a new pattern of the same substance." The nurse stays clear and *waits* in the resonating process while attending to the explications (words, colors, skin, muscles, breathing, messages, images, spirit) of the client. Moving apart occurs when the client is able to center without being connected to the nurse. This occurs gradually as the client and nurse move apart, then reconnect and move apart again, repeating the process until the client can see clearly.

Quinn's reconceptualization of therapeutic touch depicts a shared consciousness: "the pattern, or vibration of the nurse's consciousness becomes a tuning fork, resonating at a healing frequency, while the client has the opportunity within the mutual person-environment process to tune, to resonate, to that frequency" (Quinn, 1992, p. 29). Quinn points out that in a paradigm of interconnectedness, one's consciousness is integral with all consciousness; the old idea of energy exchange no longer applies because there is no here or there.

Litchfield's (1993) relationships to families who were experiencing frequent illnesses and hospitalizations of toddlers elaborates the patterning of coming together and moving apart of the nurse and client. She elicited the families' patterns by having them tell their story of what they had experienced in regard to their children's illness and hospitalization; however, it was not the content of the patterns that was the important finding of her research. It was the process whereby she as nurse-researcher entered into the family process and was able to facilitate their potential for action. She saw this process as involving: (1) a moment of partnership, (2) evolving dialogue, (3) recognizing pattern, (4) expanding horizon, and (5) increasing connectedness.

A moment of partnership was the relationship between the nurse and the client that was demarcated by their initial meeting and agreement regarding expectations of the relationship and the closure, which occurred when the client was able to see and act on their potential for action. The timing of the partnership occurred during a period of disruption characterized by uncertainty and unpredictability. The ending of the partnership occurred when the family was able to move from relative disorder to order at a higher level.

An *evolving dialogue* characterized the flow of the enfolding-unfolding process of the story of the family's life, including the researcher's participation and the wider social and political context. The differential contributions of each of the spouses and the researcher's (embodied theory) participation were elements in the dialogue, as well as the social expectations for parenting and gender roles. *Recognizing pattern* occurred as "incidental revelations" in the process of dialogue and manifested itself as changes in actions such as in movement patterns within the family and in relation to the community, expanded horizons, and increased connectedness.

The families moved from a present without vision to the presence of both past and future in a vision of possibilities. The present without vision was a kind of treadmill experience of survival without connection to the past or the future. Through the reflective process of the dialogue, they were able to envision an *expanding horizon* with plans for the future and intentions to act. In addition they were able to look beyond their own situation to what they could contribute to the larger community. The previous concentration on the child, the designated patient, was broadened to an integrated pattern of connectedness within the family and with the wider world (Litchfield, 1993)—a process of expanding consciousness.

Schubert's findings in her study of the nurse-client relationship emphasized the mutual connectedness of the nurse and client, a union based on knowing each other, caring on the part of the nurse, and trusting on the part of the client. She saw the relationship as progressing from trusting to joining to bonding, without which there was no opportunity for a working relationship (Schubert, 1989).

A similar process was identified in Lamb and Stempel's (1994) study of clients' experiences of working with a nurse case manager. They coined the term "insider-expert" to describe the role of the nurse. Vital to this role is the client's confidence in the nurse's knowledge of the medical-physiological crisis being experienced by the client and at the same time the intimacy characterized by the client's feeling of being really known and cared for by the nurse.

> Initially, clients see the nurse case manager in the role of expert, someone who can monitor their physical status and teach them ways to take care of themselves. Over time, bonding occurs between nurse and client which allows the client to feel known and cared about as an individual. In the context of this bonding, clients begin to think differently about their situations, develop confidence in their ability to care for themselves and take on greater responsibility . . . (Lamb & Stempel, 1994, p. 9)

As the client's situation stabilizes, the focus shifts to emotional and spiritual concerns and the meaning of family patterns in relation to their health. The combination of knowledge of interventions and relevance to the pattern of the person makes the difference in meaningfulness to the client. The presence and accessibility of the nurse provides consistency and support as the clients face the unpredictability of their situations.

> [Clients] state that experiencing the [nurse] case managers' concern for them helped them to think and feel differently about themselves and their situation. Individuals who had seen themselves as worthless or helpless redefined themselves as competent and valuable. [Clients] who once had viewed their current situation as unmanageable and hopeless now saw it as manageable and full of options. (Lamb & Stempel, p. 10)

This situation is illustrative of bringing order out of chaos and light out of darkness. One client described the experience of having the nurse "pull her out of a dark hole" (pp. 10-11).

The process of the clients' ability to feel competent to manage their situations on their own occurs in the post-acute phase, as the nurse provides a kind of safety net while clients try out new ways of thinking and acting and have more energy to identify their own patterns and choices. It highlights the need for the nurse to maintain the relationship with the clients across settings and over time until they are ready to stand on their own.

Similarly Litchfield's experience of the nurse's hanging in there through this process convinced her of the necessity for what Heron (1988, p. 52) has described as a "collapse into confusion, uncertainty, ambiguity, disorder and chaos . . . feeling lost to a greater or lesser degree," and tolerance for finding no outcome in the present. A reminder is helpful that order will emerge from the chaos.

Lamb and Stempel (1994) observed that clients with greater perceived need and greater comfort with intimacy seem to move through the nurse-client process of bonding, working, and changing more rapidly and with greater intensity. In contrast, the conditions described by Mishel (1990) as blocking the growth opportunities emerging from uncertainty include the clients' delayed response to their diagnosis and isolation from social interaction. These findings help to explain why some clients, whose patterns depict denial of their disease and isolation from others (Jonsdottir, *in progress*), do not manifest behaviors associated with expanding consciousness.

The way in which nursing theory is applied is by virtue of the transformation that is taking place in the person of the nurse. The transformation constitutes the nurse's field and through the interpenetration of the nurse-client field, it becomes the client's field. Whatever transforms you, transforms your practice.

Chapter Eight

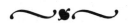

From Old Paradigm To New

As a consumer of health care services, I have often bemoaned the fact that I do not have a nurse to call my own. I have a physician and a dentist, and from time to time, a homeopath, chiropractor and massage therapist, . . . but no nurse. I know where to turn for nursing consultation because I have friends who are nurses, but until recently there has been no readily available direct access to nurses as professional practitioners. Obviously other people have resorted to the same tactics in finding a nurse because many of my nurse friends are busy helping relatives and friends (and friends of relatives and friends) who are in the midst of a health care crisis. Why are nurses not more accessible?

For the most part, historically, nursing has been caught in the bind of a subordinate role within the hospital bureaucratic structure, serving the organizational needs of hospital administration and the medical directives of physicians. Caring for patients' needs as human beings who are at some sort of health juncture in their lives—the original and primary *raison d'etre* of nursing—progressively has been squeezed out of the system by the priorities of the medical and bureaucratic establishment in providing efficient and cost-effective medical services.

DEVELOPMENT OF THE PROFESSION

Understanding of the cycles of growth of an organization (Ainsworth-Land, 1982; Land, 1973) has been helpful to me in evaluating the development of nursing as a profession. The first stage is characterized by formative activity. The phenomenon is in the process of becoming itself and establishing its identity. In nursing, as in medicine, early practitioners functioned primarily as solo practitioners in the home, a health-care situation in which there was a person-to-person relationship for the purpose of nurturing the client. Individual practitioners were in control of and responsible for their practice. Change in this stage is accretive, i.e., it expands itself and becomes more of itself.

The second stage of development is characterized as normative, a stage in which the system in interaction with the environment loses some of the authority and expansion of the first stage and develops a competitive, persuasive stance in trying to establish and maintain its own territory. Nurses, in response to rapid developments in medical technology and emphasis on hospital care, moved into the hospital setting, becoming employees of the hospital (rather than professionals relating directly to the client) and subordinates of medicine. Fragmentation and loss of continuity occurred. Hospital nursing was separated from home care nursing. Nurses began a long period of filling in the gap of medical technology, serving the needs of the bureaucratic institution and at the same time trying to fulfill nursing's original commitment of one-to-one care of persons who were ill. The demand for hospital care increased, and in order to get all the tasks completed, they were doled out as tasks per se: medicines to be distributed, blood pressures to be taken, and so on. Nurses began to lose the essence of nursing, the personalized care of earlier days.

In the third stage of growth, the integrative stage, the system begins to relate to other systems in a cooperative, mutual way. A partnership approach becomes the predominant way of life. Sometimes in this stage change takes place very rapidly; persons involved fear the loss of their previous secure status, and they seek to move "back to basics," rather than onward in the evolutionary cycle of transformation (Ainsworth-Land, 1982). There was a rather short-lived effort to go beyond the functional delivery of care to a more integrated team approach of combining individual, personalized care with some functional assignments: the concept of team nursing introduced in the early sixties. However, medicine was not partner to this approach, and the concept never really became a reality. Stage two participants are very reluctant to relinquish the territory they have gained in order to establish a cooperative approach. It was difficult to shift from a hierarchical approach to incorporate the idea that clients had to be viewed as whole persons and that the staff, in order to not be fragmented and alienated by their work, had to be fully cognizant of how their responsibilities contributed to the whole of the care for clients.

Primary nursing was a "back to basics" attempt to reestablish personal responsibility on the part of the nurse in direct relationship to the client. However, the organization of practice has not addressed the objective of ongoing professional responsibility of the nurse for the client's care over time (and across settings). Generally the primary nurse is still bound in time-space to the particular period of hospitalization in question, to the particular institution of employment, and to fulfilling at least partially the routine responsibilities of delegated medical care. As we move into the integrative stage of our development as a profession, the structure of our practice must provide for the nurse to function as a full partner in health care.

THE GAP IN HEALTH CARE

The bulk of nursing services, however, continues to be framed within and dominated by the medical model of health care (Newman & Autio, 1986; Real Nurses, 1993; Schlotfeldt, 1987). Nurses engaged in this mode of practice, albeit conscientious and dedicated, are contributing their services primarily to the implementation of medical care. This well-intended emphasis leaves the contribution to nursing care wanting. The following situation, told to me by the client, illustrates the gap in health care:

Mr. X., an 89-year-old man, lived at home with his wife of approximately the same age. He had two adult children, a son and a daughter, who was a nurse. While the daughter was out of town, Mr. X. experienced some symptoms of a stroke but was not incapacitated. The next day he fell. The son called the clinic and they instructed him to bring his father to the hospital outpatient department. Diagnostic tests confirmed the stroke, but the physician said there was nothing to be done and that the family should take "good care" of him at home. When the daughter returned, almost a week later, she noticed that Mr. X. was having difficulty with his speech, memory loss, and difficulty walking. He was eating often, sleeping, and very thirsty. She wondered if his diabetes was out of control.

The daughter called the physician, but the response was that she was "handling things fine." Her father became increasingly thirsty, irritable, hungry, and weak. Finally she felt she could not manage. She was sure his diabetes was out of control and that he was critically ill. He had Cheynes-Stokes respirations, incontinence, and was drinking gallons of water. She did not get any help with the situation until she burst into tears over the telephone and declared she absolutely could not handle the situation. The clinic staff were on strike at that time and she was told to take her father to the emergency room. There they confirmed her observations and determined that Mr. X. had a blood sugar of 700 (normal 80–120). He was admitted to the hospital in a confused, weakened state but responded immediately to the administration of insulin, bringing his blood sugar down to 400. His daughter was told that he could go home in 2–3 days, and they had a nutritionist instruct him about his diet while he was still confused. The daughter insisted she could not care for him at home, that he was too confused and weak.

Eventually a representative of the HMO (of which Mr. X. was a member) helped her explore transfer to a VA hospital. This was accomplished in approximately 12 hours. But her father was not a medical challenge, and his illness was not a service disability, and the VA agents wanted him transferred to another facility. The physician turned his case over to a social worker for placement in a nursing home. After two weeks, he was transferred to a VA-approved nursing home, for which the VA would pay for six months.

The daughter had questions about his care at the VA, but felt she had to be careful what she complained about because she didn't want to preclude his returning there if it became necessary. She felt that placing her father in the nursing home was not well thought out in terms of his particular needs. He was placed on a semi-skilled nursing unit but needed very little care—primarily food and time orientation. She observed that the people in the various organizations that treated her father—the HMO, the VA (federal system), and the nursing home (state system)—did not know what services were available in the other systems. She felt that there was no one to guide them (the patient and family) through the maze from hospital to VA to nursing home.

In the meantime the daughter was taking care of her mother, who was then living alone but did not want to leave her home. The mother was legally blind, suffered from a Parkinsonian-like tremor, and was very weak (weighing less than 90 pounds).

At the end of all this, the daughter was still worrying about whether or not she should try to bring her father home. That was what her mother wanted, but her own energy was depleted and she herself was suffering from tachycardia and osteoarthritis of the spine. Her final remark was "I have to put it all together for myself and my husband and my parents."

This situation illustrates dramatically a need that a professional nurse could answer by recognizing the seriousness of the situation and supporting the family in finding the most appropriate actions to be taken.

AN INTEGRATIVE MODEL

Fortunately things are changing. As nursing moves into the integrative stage of its development, a partnership approach becomes the predominant way of life. The system incorporates the best from previous stages. For nursing, this process involves the synthesis of individualized, intuitive caring of the formative stage of the profession's development with the medical knowledge and management skills of its normative stage into a nursing model that integrates caring, medical technology, and organizational skill in a totally new view of health and health care (Newman, 1990b).

The professional responsibilities of nursing practice include establishing a primary relationship with the client for the purpose of identifying health care needs and facilitating the clients' action potential and decision-making ability. It involves communication and collaboration with other nurses and associates in various settings where the client is being served, and collaboration with other health professionals to facilitate the client's access to needed resources. The structure of the practice is that of a direct, ongoing relationship with clients as long as nursing consultation and services are needed.

This professional nursing role, which I will refer to as nursing clinician/case manager, is the *sine qua non* of the integrative model. Two other roles appear to be essential as well.

Ever since the advent of associate degree programs in nursing, we have sought to differentiate the professional from the technical role in nursing and to articulate the two. But as we have become clearer in recognizing the disciplinary paradigms that guide practice, it becomes astonishingly clear that the issue is not primarily one of professional versus technical; it is more one of *different paradigms of practice*: disease-oriented care vis-à-vis person-oriented care. The predominant practice perspective of the current "health" care system derives from the paradigm of health as the absence of disease, a paradigm in which the battle against disease is uppermost and the practice mode is one of dominance and control. The person-oriented health paradigm espoused by the nursing profession places personal meaning and quality of life at the forefront and requires a practice mode of collaboration and mutuality.

Different views of health require different types of technology. In an institution ruled by the medical paradigm, nursing activity will be primarily medical technology. *Nursing* practice (emanating from the nursing paradigm) is outside the "reality" of the prevailing paradigm and often is viewed as nonessential extras. The emphasis on cost effectiveness has accentuated the priority of the medical regimen in the delivery of care, and nursing priorities have fallen by the wayside.

Expanding corporate structures, however, now include the full spectrum of health care services and make it possible for nurses to occupy positions which span the various care settings and attend the person-oriented health needs. In such care, when nursing practice incorporates technology from both paradigms of health, it is important that we know how the paradigms interrelate.

Movement to actualize professional nursing practice now takes the form of differentiating the nursing clinician/case manager role from the staff role, with a nursing team leader, a kind of liaison nurse, in between (Newman, 1990b). The clinician/case manager role embraces the whole of the nursing paradigm; the staff role emanates primarily from the medical paradigm; and the team leader/liaison role involves an integration and coordination of the two in an individualized program of care for each client.

Differentiation of practice is both an economy measure and a quality measure. It has not been reasonable to have practitioners with different levels of preparation doing the same thing, or to require all practitioners to have the same level of preparation. The first approach underutilizes some nurses and overextends others and does not promote a collaborative partnership in practice. The latter does not take into consideration the type of education needed for the various responsibilities of nurses in health care. Distinguishing between the responsibilities that must be enacted and matching them with an appropriate educational program is cost and quality efficient and lays the groundwork for collaboration and partnership within the nursing profession.

Places like Sioux Valley Hospital in Sioux Falls, South Dakota, under the leadership of JoEllen Koerner (1992), exemplify this collaboration. Their model of practice was first based on the work of Primm (1986), who differentiated roles for the associate degree and baccalaureate degree graduates based on level of complexity of the care involved. Subsequent evaluation of the implementation of a modified version of this model and consideration of other models of differentiation (Newman, 1990b) have led to changes in their model of differentiated practice, and now includes the clinician/case manager level of practice, which is generally agreed to require a postgraduate level of education.[1]

---

[1]Even though master's preparation for the clinical specialist/case manager role dominates the educational scene, my choice for professional education for nursing is a professional doctoral degree, the Doctor of Nursing (ND). It requires a strong arts and sciences background as pre-professional education, provides professional education comparable to that of the other major players in the health field, and brings to the program students with added personal maturity. A curriculum for such a program is not a transference of typical baccalaureate curricula in nursing to the post-graduate level. It is a new product based on the tenets of a unitary-transformative paradigm. A number of ND programs currently exist. The biggest stumbling block, as I see it, is current nursing licensure, since licensure examinations have been developed from the medical paradigm and address practice emanating from that model.

Collaboration between practitioners and educators has become a reality as we agree on the role differences in the integrated model. The nursing leaders at Sioux Valley Hospital have become partners with the educators of Augustana College and the University of South Dakota in the development of a collaborative teaching-learning-practice project called The Healing Web (Bunkers et al., 1992; Koerner & Bunkers, 1994). This project integrates the teaching of three levels of education within a practice setting that differentiates and integrates the practice of the graduates of the respective programs. The Healing Web is being implemented by nursing colleagues across the nation and is working to assure nursing's involvement in the interdisciplinary collaboration needed in order to address the health care needs of society.

NURSE CASE MANAGEMENT

Around 1985 a number of people recognized the unmet needs of clients for observation, guidance, and support beyond the walls of the hospital. Prominent among the innovators of nurse case management (NCM) is Phyllis Ethridge, at Carondelet St. Mary's Health Center in Tucson. Ethridge's program has made it possible for nurses to function to their fullest potential, free from space-time restrictions of the established hospital organization, and free to exercise their nursing judgment regarding the ongoing needs of clients in chronic, high-risk situations (Rusch, 1986). The NCM group at St. Mary's has demonstrated the cost-effectiveness of the program and contracted with an HMO in the area to provide services for their high-risk elderly clients (Ethridge, 1991; Ethridge &

Lamb, 1989; Michaels, 1991). They have become an international demonstration and consultation center for nurse case management as a model for professional nursing practice.

The role of the nurse case manager at St. Mary's exemplifies an integrated stage of professional nursing and emanates from a philosophical/theoretical base consistent with the unitary-transformative paradigm. The nurse's *relationship* with the client is paramount; it is characterized by compassion, continuity, and respect for the client's choice. Recognition of the client's life pattern over time, and unconditional acceptance of it, are important factors in identifying and respecting the client's choices. The timing of when to connect and when to separate are important factors in the effectiveness of the nursing care and are studied carefully in each nurse-client relationship. The opening of self to the client is at the heart of the relationship and is essential to the mutual growth of client and nurse for a unitary, transformative relationship to occur (Newman, Lamb & Michaels, 1992).

These dimensions of the nurse-client relationship are illustrative of elements of theory of nursing from the standpoint of health as expanding consciousness: "(1) the nurse coming together with clients at critical choice points in their lives and participating with them in the process of expanding consciousness; (2) rhythmicity and timing in the relationship; (3) letting go of the need to direct the relationship; (4) pattern identification as an essential element in the process; and (5) personal transformation" (Newman, Lamb & Michaels, 1992). These nurses had not set out to apply this theory. Their practice was an explication of the theory. Moccia (1986, p. 35), emphasizing the interdependence of theory and practice, pointed out that "theory affirms in words what practice displays in effective action."

BECOMING PARTNERS

An important aspect of the effectiveness of NCM is the coordination of the responsibilities of the nurse case manager with those of nurses working in the acute care center and in other agencies within the community. The integrative model calls for non-hierarchical relationships in which we are partners with each other, with our clients, and with other health professionals.

Bohm (1992), in the last years of his life, devoted his writing and speaking to the concept of dialogue. He saw dialogue as the means whereby we become partners, on both the local and global level. The origin of the word dialogue is "meaning flowing through." The idea of a dialogue group is to bring together 20 to 40 people from different backgrounds with different viewpoints to share their perspectives until the many incoherent thoughts become one coherent thought. This coherent thought, according to Bohm, is as powerful as a laser beam and can be envisioned circling the globe, intersecting with the beams from other groups until we reach a situation of global enlightenment.

The process of the dialogue group is different from our usual experience of group discussions, since the intent is to attend to but not defend the various thoughts set forth for consideration. Bohm points out that the word "discussion" comes from the same root as percussion and connotes a kind of batting around of ideas, rather than *receiving* of ideas as is implied in the definition, "meaning flowing through."

The council process that comes from the Native American tradition may be used to get the group started. An object that is meaningful to the group is used as "the talking stick" and only the person holding the talking stick may speak. Group members are exhorted to be honest, be brief, and to listen with their heart. This means trying not to be preoccupied with what they will say when they receive the talking stick. It is a lesson in listening and in speaking from the center of your truth. This process serves also to get all the thoughts out on the table. The story is told of a tribe who sat around for a long period of time talking until at some unpredictable point they all arose and went out, each knowing what the conclusion was without anyone having to announce it. The dialogue group is instructed not to allow itself to become goal- or task-oriented as in action groups, as that will close off a large spectrum of what is present in the group for exploration. Bohm suggests meeting regularly (just how often is optional) for approximately a year. It takes commitment on the part of the participants for the process to evolve.

The Healing Web uses this process for portions of its meetings. I have met with two other nursing groups on a monthly basis for approximately six months and found it meaningful for those who participated (many do not want this kind of intense "speaking from the heart" activity), but also difficult to maintain without some sort of established goal. Nurses tend to be action-oriented persons. We may need greater heterogeneity in the group to render it more a microcosm of the macrocosm to which we wish to generalize. Or is it possible that we may come to a point of coherent thought more quickly?

The tetra group[2] described previously (Newman, 1986a) has proved to be a meaningful way to initiate this kind of dialogue and at the same time to carry out self- or teacher-assigned

---

[2]A group of four people formed for various purposes: to just speak and listen from the heart, to pursue a learning activity, to accomplish a task.

tasks. When we first started it, we did so for self-expression and support. Our foursome was formed serendipitously of individuals with very different information-processing styles (Hermann, 1981), and we learned a lot about ourselves and our ability to work with each other. Hermann pointed out that a group made up of four different brain dominance types constitutes a "whole brain," the name of his organization, and will be more creative than a group composed of like types. With my holistic view of things, I am uncomfortable talking about a group of people making up a whole brain (Does that not imply that each of us is a part brain?), but I have experienced, both as a participant and in watching other groups operate, the value of the heterogeneity and complexity created by the interpenetration of such fields.

Tetra groups are learning groups. Nelson (1993–94) has created tetra groups in one of the courses she teaches and has found it to be so facilitative of learning that she has extended the application to the task of taking the examination. What a wonderful way to teach collaboration and partnership!

HEALTH CARE REFORM

New Zealand was and is in the midst of health care reform, and nursing leaders there have been intent on making sure that nursing assumes its rightful place in the new health care delivery system. The availability of international videoconferencing made it possible for instantaneous consultation between New Zealand nurses and nurses in the United States on the progress we are making in case management and differentiated practice. Under the leadership of Merian Litchfield (Litchfield et al., 1993), they subsequently developed a pilot project to introduce a family nurse (FN) to work with families with complex health care needs whenever and wherever their needs arise across settings and sectors. The goal was to address the need for better integration, more continuity and cost-containment in health care, and to attend to the human predicaments faced by these families. This nursing role exemplified the responsibilities of the nursing clinician/case manager and complemented the practice of other nurses in settings with a more specific focus. The theoretical foundation stemmed from Litchfield's explication of the patterning process in expanding consciousness (Litchfield, 1993). There was great satisfaction with the effectiveness of this family nurse, by the families served, the nurse herself, and other nurses involved in the care. The practice of the FN is characterized by a professional partnership with families who are "in a predicament of strife" with little or no vision of how to handle their situations. The FN supports the family in assuming control over their health circumstances by seeking and using services with discernment and increasing their sense of community as family members and citizens (Litchfield et al., 1993). If this nurse case management scheme is implemented as part of the New Zealand health reform, it will establish nursing as a freestanding health service provider.

Health reform in the United States calls for more emphasis on nursing in the community. The establishment of four Federally-funded Community Nursing Organizations charts the way for nurses to fulfill their professional responsibility to clients directly. The knowledge that guides that practice must be examined carefully to make sure the practice addresses the full spectrum of the nursing discipline. In order to be sure that the nurse has the necessary knowledge and skill to carry out this responsibility, we must pursue vigorously the theoretical development of the discipline and graduate-level education for the professional.

I believe the health care system is moving from a paradigm of health as the absence of disease to one that recognizes a dynamic, evolving pattern of the whole. In the transition we will repeatedly recognize that the "old rules" are not working anymore and be compelled to seek new patterns and arenas of practice. I am very encouraged by the changes and the significant partnerships that are taking place among nurses, in practice, research, and education. We are moving from partnership on a one-to-one basis to a global network with the center always shifting. Rather than boundaries that separate countries from each other, clients from providers, providers from other providers, this network offers connectedness and unity to the complementarity of our differences. Nursing is in a position to facilitate connections that will form a world network of cooperation, collaboration, and partnership. I anticipate that by the beginning of the 21st century, our vision for nursing will be a reality.

Chapter Nine

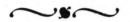

Letting Go, Moving On

It is time for
A parting with the past.
It is time to
Replace the anchor of the past
With the pull of the future.

(Newman, 1994)

We are at a breakpoint in nursing history. We have the opportunity of our professional lifetime.

My reason for entering nursing was to understand the process of health and illness, so that I could help people move through health crises. In the process of learning about health and illness, I learned techniques that were a part of medical care. It was not what I wanted to do. But I forced myself to be fairly proficient at those things in order to function as a professional nurse. As a graduate student, I wrote an essay elaborating on what I deemed the essence of nursing—love in the sense that Erich Fromm described—and I asserted that we should let go of those instrumental medical tasks that we had taken on and get on with the practice of nursing. My instructor responded, "But can we?" I felt intimidated and didn't pursue the matter further at that time.

Then a breakpoint occurred in the late sixties when the medical profession realized that they were not getting the assistance they wanted from the nursing profession and initiated a new category of worker, the physician's assistant. A graduate student again, I wrote a position paper on this new phenomenon and responded: "Yes! The physicians need assistance. Let's support this new worker, so that we can let go of those medical tasks and get on with fulfilling the purpose of our mission as a profession." A different instructor was outraged at the thought of letting go of a portion of what she regarded as nursing territory. Again I felt intimidated. I wasn't sure enough of my own judgment, and let the matter drop. I've been sorry ever since.

But now we come to this issue again. What is going to be our predominant arena of practice, medicine or nursing, or both? Perhaps what we need is not so much a rejection of those aspects of medical technology that we have taken on but a *transformation* of them within a new paradigm. Watson (1987) urges nursing to hold on to the timelessness of caring, which can transform technology and place science and technology within the context of human meaning.

We are at another breakpoint. The Nation recognizes that there is something missing in our present health care system. A person hospitalized in the current system *may* experience the efficient administration of medicine and treatments, but the human factor, the caring, is missing. And what happens once one leaves the hospital? Nursing has been making progress in preparing graduate degree nurses as independent primary care providers who are capable of providing the caring, comprehensive service needed by society, but there is still a chance that reforms in health care will take place without nurses as major players. The medical profession has taken a stand to bar nurses from serving as primary care providers. We *must not allow ourselves to become intimidated* as this opportunity presents itself to become what we can be in answering society's need.

> We are in the process of creating
> A shared vision.
> In order to do so
> It is necessary
> To connect all parts of the system,
> To integrate the similar
> And the dissimilar
> Unleashing the power of creativity.
>
> (Newman, 1994)

A paradigm shift to a collaborative caring model based on a unitary, transformative vision of health can encompass medical technology as an alternative within the whole, rather than the primary focus. A shift in paradigm does not discard the old knowledge; it transforms it by viewing it from another perspective. As we become clear on the nursing paradigm, medical technology will be transformed within the context of the whole. The practice of nursing is not, as Mechanic and Aiken (1986) so aptly stated, "the soft underbelly" of medicine but the mind and heart that makes transformation of the health experience possible. It is *caring in the human health experience*. This synthesis of the two major concepts of nursing's metaparadigm clearly distinguishes the focus of nursing from that of medicine; it encompasses the vast array of health experiences not specifically associated with disease and makes clear the profession's commitment to extend itself in service to society. The characteristics of caring emerge as ubiquitous to the effective nurse-client relationship (Butrin, 1992; Lamb & Stempel, 1994) even when we are not looking for them. The health perspective demanded by caring is one of unconditional acceptance of the pattern of the whole. The new rules call for unconditional love, which manifests itself in sensitivity to self, attention to others, and creativity. The essence of the process is in being fully present in the transformation of ourselves and others as we allow the meaning of the new reality to unfold.

The shared vision will come about through dialogue. Land and Jarman (1992) point out that organizations don't change; only individuals change, and through individuals, the pattern of the whole. This process involves knowing who you are, what you care about, what you love. The power of future pull is in knowing your purpose and vision and in bringing about circumstances in which everyone can win.

If we can accept caring in the human health experience as our focus, we know who we are, what we care about, and what we need to know. Theories of nursing, the science of nursing, must address this complex, holistic dynamic. This focus requires a scientific paradigm that embraces a unitary, transformative perspective, one in which the living system is involved in a series of giant fluctuations of unpredictable transformations. Knowledge based on objectivity and control is relevant to one phase of this process but insufficient for full elaboration and understanding of the nursing phenomenon.

CARING AS A MORAL IMPERATIVE

Care, says Thomas Moore, is what a nurse does, and soul is a dimension of experience having to do with relatedness, heart, depth, and values. Moore's description of care of the soul co-incides with what I see to be nursing's responsibility in the new paradigm:

> Care of the soul . . . isn't about curing, fixing, changing, ad-justing or making healthy . . . It doesn't look to the future for an ideal, trouble-free existence. Rather, it remains patiently in the present, close to life as it presents itself day by day . . ." (1992, p. xv)

He goes on to say that care of the soul is about attending to the decisions and changes of everyday life; it is living fully the presenting pattern rather than eliminating it as a problem. He warns that we need to resist the "savior impulse" and con-centrate on listening and looking carefully at what is being revealed in a person's suffering: "By doing less, more is ac-complished" (p. 10). A painful and seemingly impossible situ-ation is simply the complexity of human life. What is needed is "not taking sides when there is a conflict at a deep level. It may be necessary to stretch the heart wide enough to embrace contradiction and paradox" (Moore, 1992).

I believe that caring is a moral imperative for nursing. Going through the motions of job responsibilities without caring is not nursing. Theory that does not take into consid-eration the caring dimension is not nursing theory. To para-phrase Moss' statement on love, we like to think of caring as something we can do, rather than something that transforms us and all that we do. It is a reflection of the whole of oneself. This kind of caring brings forth the ugly and the lowly as well as the beautiful and the lofty. For the person who is ready, the art of caring is the deliberate loss of control: "the letting go of the obsession with self, the surrender into being, the open-ing of the heart" (Moss, 1981, pp. 10–11).

To be open is to be vulnerable, an important characteristic of humanness. To be vulnerable is often to suffer. We tend to avoid suffering, and yet avoidance of suffering may deter movement to higher levels of consciousness. Suffering offers us the opportunity to transcend a particular situation. Vulnerability, suffering, disease, death do not diminish us. What does diminish us is trying to protect ourselves by binding ourselves off from these experiences. The need is to let go, embrace our experience, and allow the expansion of consciousness to unfold.

Epilogue
A Dialogue with John Heron

John Heron's work on cooperative inquiry was influential in the development of a method of inquiry suitable to the theory of health as expanding consciousness. In the spring of 1992 I sent Dr. Heron a copy of the 1986 version of *Health as Expanding Consciousness*. His questions in response were provocative and helped me to clarify where this theory was leading nursing as a profession. Therefore I have included some of his questions and my answers (as elaborated in correspondence between the two of us in April and May of 1992) in the hope that this dialogue will be helpful to the reader.

Heron: If health is the integration of disease and non-disease in an expansion of consciousness, then (a) does the client's expansion through mental/behavioral/situational change cure the disease, thus rendering most of physical medicine irrelevant; or (b) is physical medicine just an external addition to the client's integration and expansion process; or is it sometimes (a) and sometimes (b), in which case how do you know which of them is appropriate?

143

Newman: I see the paradigm in which the theory of expanding consciousness fits as encompassing the view of health represented by physical medicine but not dominated by it. It is possible for a person to move to another level of consciousness at which the disease can be relinquished (as the system's way of manifesting its pattern), but if this is not possible, the expansion occurs through the experience of the disease. It is not a matter of either/or. The process of expanding consciousness is ongoing, regardless of the circumstances, and one may choose to accept or not accept the physical medicine approach, depending on personal perspective and available information.

Heron: If (b) is the case and medical intervention is a part of the expansion process, then doesn't the physical medicine of doctors become subordinate to the primary care of the nurse as you define it? Is not the nurse the one who should be the prime facilitator of the expansion process, and who should alert the doctor to his or her role in that overall process?

Newman: Yes, I agree with your interpretation. The nurse has a more holistic view of the client's health experience than the very circumscribed treatment-of-disease approach. I have been working with a group of nurses in Tucson, Arizona who are functioning in the way you describe.

Heron: If this is so, then how can your model ever be properly applied and given the chance it deserves in the current hospital system, where the physical medicine model controls and limits nursing through doctor dominance?

Newman: It is not possible to adequately apply my model in the hospital situation, not only because of the dominance of the physical medicine regimen, but also because of the cost factor. Hospitals are being run as businesses, which must make a profit, and that is done by making sure that all of the medical orders are done quickly and efficiently. This means there is little or no time for individual, interpersonal, caring relationships between client and nurse. The nurses I refer to function as case managers (not a good term for nursing practice because we do not think of our clients as "cases" and the philosophy of this theory is partnership, not management, but nevertheless the term has been used) in direct relationship to the clients *wherever* and *whenever* the clients have need for assistance in their own health care. Their practice is very consistent with my model.

Heron: Does a healthy expanded consciousness (HEC), (a) mean the end, resolution and cure of the disease; or (b) does it only mean integrating the continuing disease process in a whole new way of being (so a person can be completely healthy in terms of an expanded consciousness even though they still have cancer); or is it sometimes (a) and in other cases (b), in which case how do you tell when HEC is met by the one or the other?

Newman: The process of expanding consciousness is not healthy or unhealthy. It simply *is*. My experience with the process has been primarily the way you describe in (b), the integration of disease, but it is possible for the person to transcend the disease. Richard Moss cites instances of transcending the disease process in his books. There is no standard to be met in terms of "healthy expanded consciousness." The process is ongoing, and each person is at a different level (or perhaps, different point in space-time).

Appendix

Protocol for Research on
Health as Expanding Consciousness

The data collection process entails one initial interview of 45–60 minutes focused on what is most meaningful in the experience of the participant(s). After the initial pattern analysis, as described below, one or more subsequent interviews are conducted to reflect on the pattern depicted in the data. Each interview is tape recorded. The steps in the process are as follows:

1. **The Interview:** After explanation of the study and agreement of the participant to continue, the initial interview begins with a simple, open-ended statement such as: "Tell me about the most meaningful persons and events in your life." (This question may be modified to fit the particular focus of the study.) The interview proceeds in a non-directive manner. If the interviewee needs help in thinking of something considered important, the interviewer may prompt the interviewee to think of something from childhood that stands out in memory.

   The interviewer is an active listener and clarifies and reflects as necessary. The interviewer is free to disclose aspects of him- or herself that are deemed appropriate. Occasionally more direct questions are utilized. In being fully present in the moment, the interviewer will be sensitive to intuitive hunches about what to say or ask.

2. **Transcription:**   Soon after the interview is completed, the interviewer listens carefully to and transcribes the tape. There are times when the interviewee will get off on a topic that does not relate directly to his life pattern (e.g., the details of a recipe, or some other aside). The interviewer will be sensitive to the relevance of the data and may omit it in the transcription (with an appropriate note to the place on the tape in case it later seems important).

3. **Development of Narrative:**   The interviewer selects the statements deemed most important to the interviewee and arranges the key segments of the data in chronological order to highlight the most significant events and persons. The data remains the same except in the order of presentation. Natural breaks where a pattern shift occurs are noted and form the basis of the sequential patterns. The pattern of the whole will emerge, made up of segments of the interviewee's relationships over time.

4. **Diagram:**   The narrative is then transmuted into a simple diagram of the sequential pattern configurations. This step is optional but has been found helpful in actually seeing the pattern of the whole.

5. **Follow-up:**   In the second interview, the diagram (or other visual portrayal) is shared with the interviewee. No interpretation is made. This is simply an illustration of the participant's story in graphic form, which tends to accentuate the contrasts or repetitions in relationships over time. This mutual viewing is an opportunity for the interviewee to confirm and clarify or revise the story being portrayed. If the interviewer is in doubt about any aspect of the story, now is the time to clarify.

The nature of the pattern of person-environment interaction will begin to emerge in terms of the energy flow, e.g., blocked, diffuse, disorganized, repetitive, or whatever descriptors and metaphors come to mind to describe the pattern. The interviewee may express signs that pattern recognition is occurring (or has already occurred in the interval following the first interview) as the interviewee and interviewer reflect together on the interviewee's life pattern. If not, either of the participants may want to proceed with additional reflections in subsequent interviews until no further insight is reached. Sometimes no signs of pattern recognition emerge, and if so, that characterizes the pattern for that person. It is not to be forced.

6. **Application of the Theory:** After the interviews are completed, more intense analysis of the data is undertaken by the investigator in light of the theory of expanding conociousness. The nature of the sequential patterns of interaction are evaluated in terms of quality and complexity and interpreted according to the participant's position on Young's spectrum of consciousness. They represent presentational relationships (see Chapter 6, pp. 88–92). Similarities of pattern among participants of the study may be designated by themes and stated in propositional form.

Bibliography

Ainsworth-Land, G. (1984). *New rules for growth and change.* Eden Prairie, MN: Wilson Learning Corporation.

Ainsworth-Land, G., & V.((1982). *Forward to basics.* Buffalo: D.O.K.

Allport, G. (1961). *Pattern and growth in personality.* New York: Holt, Rinehart & Winston.

Antonovsky, A. (1979). *Health, stress and coping.* San Francisco: Jossey-Bass.

Ardell, D. B. (1977). *High level wellness.* Emmaus, PA: Rodale Press.

Arguelles, J. (1987). *Mayan New Year* (Audiotape). The Santa Fe event. Santa Fe: Doorways.

Bateson, G. (1979). *Mind and nature: A necessary unity.* Toronto: Bantam.

Bentov, I. (1978). *Stalking the wild pendulum.* New York: E. P. Dutton.

Bohm, D. (1980). *Wholeness and the implicate order.* London: Routledge & Kegan Paul.

Bohm, D. (1981). The physicist and the mystic—is a dialogue between them possible? A conversation with David Bohm conducted by Renee Weber. *Re-Vision*, 4(1), 22–35.

Bohm, D. (1992). On dialogue. *Noetic Sciences Review*, No. 23, 16–18.

Bramwell, L. (1984). Use of the life history in pattern identification and health promotion. *Advances in Nursing Science*, 7(1), 37–44.

Brodsky, A. B. (1986). The manners of chaos: A conversation between W. McWhinney and D. Dunn. *International Synergy*, 1, 40–51.

Bunkers, S., Brendtro, M., Holmes, P., Howell, J., Johnson, S., Koerner, J., Larson, J., Nelson, J., & Weaver, R. (1992). The healing web, a transformative model of nursing. *Nursing & Health Care*, 13(2), 68–73.

Butrin, J. (1992). Cultural diversity in the nurse-client encounter. *Clinical Nursing Research*, 1(3), 238–251.

Capra, F. (1982). *The turning point*. New York: Simon & Schuster.

Condon, W. S. (1980). The relation of interactional synchrony and cognitive and emotional processes. In M. R. Key (Ed.), *The relationship of verbal and nonverbal communication*. New York: Mouton Publishing, pp. 48–65.

Cowles, K. V. (1988). Personal world expansion for survivors of murder victims. *Western Journal of Nursing Research*, 10(6), 687–698.

Cunningham, A. J. (1993). Does cancer have "meaning"? *Advances, The Journal of Mind-Body Health*, 9(1), 63–69.

Davis, M. (1982). *Interaction rhythms: Periodicity in communicative behavior*. New York: Human Sciences.

Dolfman, M. L. (1973). The concept of health: An historic and analytic examination. *Journal of School Health, 43,* 491–497.

Dossey, L. (1982). *Space, time, and medicine.* Boulder: Shambhala.

Dossey, L. (1984). *Beyond illness: Discovering the experience of health.* Boulder: Shambhala.

Dubos, R. (1965). *Man adapting.* New Haven: Yale University Press.

Dunn, H. L. (1959). High-level wellness for man and society. *American Journal of Public Health, 49,* 786–792.

Dunn, H. L. (1973). *High level wellness.* Arlington, VA: Beatty.

Engle, V. F. (1984). Newman's conceptual framework and the measurement of older adults' health. *Advances in Nursing Science, 7*(1), 2–36.

Engle, V. F. (1985). The relationship of movement and time to older adults' functional health. *Research in Nursing and Health, 9,* 123–129.

Ethridge, P. (1991). A nursing HMO: Carondelet St. Mary's experience. *Nursing Management, 22*(7), 22–27.

Ethridge, P., & Lamb, G. S. (1989). Professional nursing case management improves quality, access and costs. *Nursing Management, 20*(3), 30–35.

Ferguson, M. (1980). *The aquarian conspiracy: Personal and social transformation in the 1980s.* Los Angeles: J. P. Tarcher.

Friedman, H. L. (1983). The self-expansiveness level form: A conceptualization and measurement of a transpersonal construct. *The Journal of Transpersonal Psychology, 15,* 37–50.

Fryback, P. B. (1993). Health for people with a terminal diagnosis. *Nursing Science Quarterly, 6*(3), 147–159.

Fuller, R. B. (1975). *Synergetics.* New York: Macmillan.

Gendlin, E. T. (1978). *Focusing.* New York: Everest.

Gottlieb, R. (1982). *The eye gym and the power to know.* Power of Knowing Conference, Berkeley, CA, May 25–27.

Grof, S. (1985). *Beyond the brain.* Albany, NY: State University of New York Press.

Guba, E. G., & Lincoln, Y. S. (1989). *Fourth generation evaluation.* Newbury Park, CA: Sage.

Hall, E. T. (1984). *The dance of life: The other dimension of time.* Garden City, NY: Anchor/Doubleday.

Hall, R. L., & Cobey, V. E. (1974). The world as crystallized movement. *Main Currents, 31*(1), 4–7.

Hart, L. A. (1978). The new "brain" concept of learning. *Phi Delta Kappan,* February, 393–396.

Hermann, N. (1981). The creative brain. *Training and Development Journal, 35,* 10–16.

Heron, J. (1981). Philosophical basis for a new paradigm. In P. Reason & J. Rowan (Eds.), *Human inquiry: A sourcebook of new paradigm research.* New York: Wiley, pp. 19–35.

Heron, J. (1988). Validity in co-operative inquiry. In P. Reason (Ed.), *Human inquiry in action: Developments in new paradigm research.* London: Sage, pp. 40–59.

Jantsch, E. (1980). *The self-organizing universe.* New York: Pergamon.

Jones, R. S. (1982). *Physics as metaphor.* New York: Meridian.

Jonsdottir, H. (In progress). *Life patterns of people with chronic obstructive pulmonary disease.* PhD dissertation, University of Minnesota, Minneapolis, MN.

Keen, S. (1978). Self-love and the cosmic connection. *Re-Vision, 1*(3/4), 88–89.

Koerner, J. G. (1992). Differentiated practice: the evolution of professional nursing. *Journal of Professional Nursing, 8,* 335–341.

Koerner, J. G., Bunkers, L. B., Nelson, B., & Santema, K. (1989). Implementing differentiated practice: The Sioux Valley Hospital experience. *Journal of Nursing Administration, 19*(2), 13–22.

Koerner, J. G., & Bunkers, S. S. (1994). The healing web. An expansion of consciousness. *Journal of Holistic Nursing, 12*(1), 51–63.

Lamb, G. S., & Stempel, J. E. (1994). Nurse case management from the client's view: Growing as insider-expert. *Nursing Outlook, (42),* 7–13.

Lamendola, F., & Newman, M. A. (1994). The paradox of HIV/AIDS as expanding consciousness. *Advances in Nursing Science, 16*(3), 13–21.

Land, G. T. L. (1973). *Grow or die.* New York: Dell.

Land, G., & Jarman, B. (1992). *Breakpoint and beyond.* New York: HarperBusiness.

Lather, P. (1986). Research as praxis. *Harvard Educational Review, 56*(3), 257–277.

Leonard, G. (1978). *The silent pulse.* New York: E. P. Dutton.

Lerner, M., & Remen, R. N. (1985). Varieties of integral cancer therapies. *Advances, 2* (3), 14–33.

LeShan, L. (1989). Cancer as a turning point. *Noetic Sciences Review,* (11), 22–28.

Litchfield, M. C. (1993). *The process of health patterning in families with young children who have been repeatedly hospitalized.* Master's thesis, University of Minnesota, Minneapolis, MN.

Litchfield, M., Connor, M., Eathorne, T., Laws, M., McCombie, M-L., & Smith, S. (1993). *Direction for nursing practice and service delivery in the New Zealand health reforms.* Report of the pilot study of the Wellington professional nurse case management project. Wellington, New Zealand.

Marchione, J. M. (1986). Application of the new paradigm of health to individuals, families, and communities. In M. Newman, *Health as expanding consciousness.* St. Louis: Mosby.

Martin, M. (1985). Letter to author, 13 November 1985.

Mechanic, D., & Aiken, L. H. (1986). Social science, medicine and health policy. In L. H. Aiken and D. Mechanic (Eds.), *Applications of social science to clinical medicine and health policy.* New Brunswick, NJ: Rutgers University Press.

Meleis, A. (1993). A passion for substance revisited: global transitions and international commitments. *Proceedings of the 1993 Annual Forum on Doctoral Nursing Education.* Minneapolis: University of Minnesota School of Nursing.

Mentzer, C., & Schorr, J. A. (1986). Perceived situational control and perceived duration of time: Expressions of life patterns. *Advances in Nursing Science, 9*(1), 12–20.

Michaels, C. (1991). A nursing HMO—Ten months with Carondelet St. Mary's Hospital-based nurse case management. *Aspen's Advisor for Nurse Executives, 6*(11).

Mikunas, A. (1974). The primacy of movement. *Main Currents, 31*(1), 8–12.

Mishel, M. H. (1990). Reconceptualization of the uncertainty in illness theory. *Image, 22*(4), 256–261.

Moch, S. D. (1990). Health within the experience of breast cancer. *Journal of Advanced Nursing, 15,* 1426–1435.

Moccia, P. (1986). *New approaches to theory development.* New York: National League for Nursing Press.

Moore, T. (1992). *Care of the soul.* New York: HarperCollins.

Morgan, G. (1983). Toward a more reflective social science. In G. Morgan (Ed.), *Beyond method: Strategies for social research* (pp. 368–376). Beverly Hills: Sage.

Moss, R. (1981). *The I that is we.* Millbrae, CA: Celestial Arts.

Moustakas, C. (1990). *Heuristic research.* Newbury Park, CA: Sage.

Muses, C. (1978). *Higher dimensions and systems relating science and spirit.* Paper presented at symposium on New Dimensions of Consciousness, sponsored by Sufi Order in the West, New York, November 17–20.

Nelson, J. (1993–94). Personal communication.

Newman, M. A. (1972). Time estimation in relation to gait tempo. *Perceptual and Motor Skills, 34,* 359–366.

Newman, M. A. (1976). Movement tempo and the experience of time. *Nursing Research, 25,* 273–279.

Newman, M. A. (1978). *Toward a theory of health.* Paper presented at Nurse Educator Conference, New York, NY.

Newman, M. A. (1979). *Theory development in nursing.* Philadelphia: Davis.

Newman, M. A. (1982). Time as an index of expanding consciousness with age. *Nursing Research, 31,* 290–293.

Newman, M. A. (1983a). Editorial. *Advances in Nursing Science*, 5(2), x–xi.

Newman, M. A. (1983b). Newman's health theory. In I. Clements & F. Roberts (Eds.), *Family health: A theoretical approach to nursing care*. New York: Wiley, pp. 161–175.

Newman, M. A. (1984). Nursing diagnosis: Looking at the whole. *American Journal of Nursing, 84*, 1496–1499.

Newman, M. A. (1986a). *Health as expanding consciousness*. St. Louis: Mosby.

Newman, M. A. (1986b). Nursing's emerging paradigm: The diagnosis of pattern. In A. M. McLane (Ed.), *Classification of nursing diagnoses*, Proceedings of the seventh conference of the North American Nursing Diagnosis Association (pp. 53–60). St. Louis: Mosby.

Newman, M. A. (1987a). Aging as increasing complexity. *Journal of Gerontological Nursing, 13*(9), 16–18.

Newman, M. A. (1987b). Patterning. In M. Duffy & N. J. Pender (Eds.), *Conceptual Issues in Health Promotion*. A report of proceedings of a Wingspread conference. Indianapolis: Sigma Theta Tau International.

Newman, M. A. (1989). The spirit of nursing. *Holistic Nursing Practice, 3*(3), 1–6.

Newman, M. A. (1990a). Newman's theory of health as praxis. *Nursing Science Quarterly, 3*(1), 37–41.

Newman, M. A. (1990b). Toward an integrative model of professional practice. *Journal of Professional Nursing, 6*(3), 167–173.

Newman, M. A. (1992a). Health conceptualizations. In J. J. Fitzpatrick, R. L. Taunton, & A. K. Jacox (Eds.), *Annual*

Review of Nursing Research, 9, 221–243. New York: Springer.

Newman, M. A. (1992b). Prevailing paradigms in nursing. *Nursing Outlook, 40*(1), 10–14.

Newman, M. A. (1994). Into the 21st century. *Nursing Science Quarterly, 7*(1), 44–46.

Newman, M. A. (In press). Theory for nursing practice. *Nursing Science Quarterly.*

Newman, M. A., & Autio, S. (1986). Nursing in the world of DRGs and prospective payment. *CURA Reporter* (University of Minnesota Center for Urban and Regional Affairs), *16*(5), 1–7.

Newman, M. A., & Gaudiano, J. (1984). Depression as an explanation for decreased subjective time in the elderly. *Nursing Research, 33,* 137–139.

Newman, M. A., Lamb, G. S., & Michaels, C. (1992). Nursing case management: The coming together of theory and practice. *Nursing & Health Care, 12,* 404–408.

Newman, M. A., & Moch, S. D. (1991). Life patterns of persons with coronary heart disease. *Nursing Science Quarterly, 4,* 161–167.

Newman, M. A., Sime, A. M., & Corcoran-Perry, S. A. (1991). The focus of the discipline of nursing. *Advances in Nursing Science, 14*(1), 1–6.

Ostrander, S., & Schroeder, L. (1971). *Psychic discoveries behind the iron curtain.* New York: Bantam.

Parse, R. R. (1987). *Nursing science: Major paradigms, theories, and critiques.* Philadelphia: Saunders.

Parsons, T. (1958). Definitions of health and illness in the light of American values and social structure. In E. Jaco (Ed.), *Patients, physicians, and illness*. Glencoe, IL: Free Press.

Peck, M. S. (1978). *The road less travelled*. New York: Simon & Schuster.

Pelletier, K. R. (1978). *Toward a science of consciousness*. New York: Dell.

Polkinghorne, D. E. (1988). *Narrative knowing and the human sciences*. Albany, NY: State University of New York Press.

Prigogine, I. (1976). Order through fluctuation: Self-organization and social system. In E. Jantsch & C. H. Waddington (Eds.), *Evolution and Consciousness*. Reading, MA: Addison-Wesley, pp. 93–133.

Prigogine, I. (1980). *From being to becoming*. San Francisco: W. H. Freeman.

Prigogine, I., Allen, P. M., & Herman, R. (1977). Long-term trends and the evaluation of complexity. In E. Laszlo & J. Bierman (Eds.), *Goals in a global community: The original background papers for Goals for Mankind* (Vol. 1). New York: Pergamon Press, pp. 1–63.

Prigogine, I., & Stengers, I. (1984). *Order out of chaos*. Boulder: Shambhala.

Primm, P. L. (1986). Defining and differentiating ADN and BSN competencies. *Issues* (National Council of State Boards of Nursing, Inc.), 7(1), 1–6.

Quinn, J. F. (1992). Holding sacred space. The nurse as healing environment. *Holistic Nursing Practice*, 6(4), 26–36.

Real Nurses (videotape). (1993). WQED/Pittsburgh with cooperation of Allegheny General Hospital and the Volunteer Hospitals of America, Pennsylvania region.

Ravitz, L. J. (1962). History, measurement, and applicability of periodic changes in the electromagnetic field in health and disease. *Annals of the New York Academy of Science, 98*, 1144–1201.

Reed, P. G. (1991). Toward a nursing theory of self-transcendence: Deductive reformulation using developmental theories. *Advances in Nursing Science, 13* (4), 64–77.

Reynolds, C. L. (1988). The measurement of health in nursing research. *Advances in Nursing Science, 10*(4), 23–31.

Rogers, M. E. (1970). *An introduction to the theoretical basis of nursing.* Philadelphia: Davis.

Rusch, S. C. (1986). Continuity of care: From hospital unit into home. *Nursing Management, 17*(12), 38–41.

Sarter, B. (1988). Philosophic sources of nursing theory. *Nursing Science Quarterly, 1*(2), 52–59.

Schlotfeldt, R. M. (1987). Resolution of issues: An imperative for creating nursing's future. *Journal of Professional Nursing, 3*, 136–142.

Schmitt, N. A. (1991). *Caregiving couples: The experience of giving and receiving social support.* PhD dissertation, University of Minnesota, Minneapolis, MN.

Schorr, J. A. (1983). Manifestations of consciousness and the developmental phenomenon of death. *Advances in Nursing Science, 5*, 28–35.

Schorr, J. A., Farnham, R. C., & Ervin, S. M. (1991). Health patterns in aging women as expanding consciousness. *Advances in Nursing Science, 13(4)*, 52–63.

Schorr, J. A., & Schroeder, C. A. (1991). Movement and time: Exertion and perceived duration. *Nursing Science Quarterly, 4*(3), 104–112.

Schubert, P. E. (1989). *Mutual connectedness: Holistic nursing practice under varying conditions of intimacy*. PhD Dissertation. San Francisco: University of California.

Seagel, S. (1982). Auditory perspective enlarges realm of hearing. *Brain-Mind Bulletin, 8*(1), 1–2.

Sheldrake, R. (1983a). *A new science of life*. Los Angeles: Tarcher.

Sheldrake, R. (1983b). Testing a new science of life. *Investigations, 1*(1), 1–8.

Smith, A. (1975). *Powers of the mind*. New York: Random House.

Smith, C. A. (In press). The lived experience of staying healthy in rural African American families. *Nursing Science Quarterly*.

Smith, M. J. (1988). Perspectives of wholeness: The lens makes a difference. *Nursing Science Quarterly, 1*(3), 94–95.

Stephens, G. J. (1965). The time factor—should it control the patient's care? *American Journal of Nursing, 65*, 77–82.

Stone, H. (1978). *Holism: A new vision of man, a new vision of health*. Paper presented at conference on Holistic Perspectives: A Renaissance in Medicine and Health Care, Philadelphia, November 11–12.

Teilhard de Chardin, P. (1959). *The phenomenon of man*. New York: Harper & Brothers.

Thomas, L. (1979). *The medusa and the snail*. New York: Viking.

Thompson, W. I. (1986). The Sunday evening evolutionary times. *International Synergy, 1*, 21–27.

Thompson, W. I. (1989). *Imaginary landscape making worlds of myth and science*. New York: St. Martin's.

Tiller, W. A. (1973). Some energy field observations of man and nature. In S. Krippner (Ed.), *Galaxies of life*. New York: Interface, pp. 71–111.

Tommet, P. (1992). *Pattern of the person*. Unpublished manuscript. Minneapolis, MN.

Tompkins, E. S. (1980). Effect of restricted mobility and dominance on perceived duration. *Nursing Research, 29,* 333–338.

Ubell, E. (1985). A world without disease. *Parade Magazine,* January 27.

Vaill, P. B. (1984–1985). Process wisdom for a new age. *Re-Vision, 7*(2), 39–49.

Vaughan, F. E. (1979). Transpersonal dimensions of psychotherapy. *Re-Vision, 2*(1), 26–29.

Walker, L. O. (1971). Toward a clearer understanding of the concept of nursing theory. *Nursing Research, 20,* 428–435.

Watson, J. (1985). *Nursing: Human science and human care*. Norwalk: Appleton-Century-Crofts.

Watson, J. (1987). Nursing on the caring edge: Metaphorical vignettes. *Advances in Nursing Science, 10,* 10–18.

Watson, L. (1976). *Gifts of unknown things*. New York: Simon & Schuster.

Watson, L. (1978). *Evolution and the unconscious*. Paper presented at symposium on New Dimensions of Consciousness, sponsored by Sufi Order in the West, New York, November 17–20.

Weber, R. (1984). Compassion, rootedness, and detachment: Their role in healing. A conversation with Dora Kunz. *Re-Vision, 7*(1), 76–82.

West, M. C. (1984). *Patterns of health in mothers of developmentally disabled children*. Unpublished master's thesis. The Pennsylvania State University, University Park, PA.

Wheeler, C. E., & Chinn, P. L. (1984). *Peace and power: A handbook of feminist process*. Buffalo: Margaret-daughters.

Whyte, L. L. (1974). *The universe of experience*. New York: Harper & Row.

Wilber, K. (1983). *Up for Eden*. Boulder: Shambhala.

Young, A. M. (1976a). *The geometry of meaning*. San Francisco: Robert Briggs.

Young, A. M. (1976b). *The reflexive universe: Evolution of consciousness*. San Francisco: Robert Briggs.

Index

A

Absolute consciousness, 35–36, 48
AIDS. *See* HIV/AIDS, 22
Aiken L. H., 139
Ainsworth-Land, G., 47, 120
Allen, P. M., 37n, 39–40
Allport, G., 77–78
Amyotrophic lateral sclerosis, 60
Antonovsky, A., 4
Ardell, D. B., 4
Arguelles, J., 109
Augustana College, South Dakota, 128
Autio, S., 122

B

Bateson, Gregory, 72, 73, 74, 99
Bentov, I., xvii, xxv–xxvi, 29, 33, 36, 61, 66, 67
Biological rhythms, 11
Bohm, D., xxvi, 6–7, 8, 10, 36, 57, 61, 74, 83–84, 88, 106, 130

Bramwell, L., 86
Brodie, John, 61
Bunkers, S., 128
Butrin, J., 84, 140
Byers, Paul, 58–59

C

Cancer
  as consciousness, turning point in, 65–66
  as manifestation of pattern of the whole, 20, 23–24, 107–08
Capra, F., 10
Caring as moral imperative, xix, 140–42
Carondelet St. Mary's Health Center, Arizona, xvii, 128–29
Causality, 28, 62
Causation, formative, Sheldrake's hypothesis of, 40–41
Chinese medicine, 19
Chinn, P. L., 92

Choices leading to higher
levels of consciousness,
46
Chronobiology, 74–75
Circadian cycle, 53–56
Client and nurse relationship,
112–16
Cobey, V. E., 58, 59
Community and family pat-
terns of health and
disease, 25–29, 115
Community Nursing Organization, 133
Condon, W. S., 56, 84
Consciousness, 33–36
absolute, 35–36, 48
Bentov's theory of evolution
of, xxv
centers of, individual, family, and community, 24
definition of, 33–34
disorder as necessary predecessor, 47
evolution of, xxv, 34, 36–48
pattern recognition as
turning point in, 41–43,
65
expanding
concept of, 33–34, 145
health as, formulation of
concept of, xxiii–xxvi
manifestation of, 51–68
health as evolution of, 43–48
higher levels of, choices
leading to, 46
highest levels of, 66–67
kinesthetic, 57
love and, xxvi, 67
matter as manifestation of,
36

movement, integration of
via, 56–60
people as centers of, 24
and suffering, 142
time-space-movement as
manifestation of, 51–68
world, 57
Corcoran-Perry, S., xviii, 52,
82
Coronary heart disease, 20, 66,
90, 91, 92
Council process, 130–31
Cowles, K. V., 64
Cowling, R., 86
Crisis causing pattern change,
28–29
Cunningham, A. J., 65–66

D

Davis, M., 84
Deikman, A. J., 63
Diabetes, 17
Dialogue and dialogue group,
130–32, 140
Disability, developmental, 29–
30, 68
Disease
as consciousness, expand-
ing, 23–24, 65
as energy state, high, 21
and evolution of person, 21
family and community pat-
tern of, 25–29
as health, manifestation of,
5–12
heart, as manifestation of
pattern of the whole, 20
as integrating factor, 20–22
necessity of, 29–30

as pattern
  emergent, 22–23
  manifestation of, 17–22
  of person-environment in-
    teraction, 17, 44
  as process, 12
  tension characteristic of, 21–
    22
  as the whole, manifestation
    of, xvi, 7, 9
Dissipative structures, Prigo-
    gine's theory of, 37–
    40, 102 (fig.)
Doberneck, B., 104
Dolfman, M. L., 4
Dossey, L., 10, 22
Dubos, R., 4
Dunn, D., 22
Dunn, H. L., 4

E

Education, xviii, 127n, 134, 138
  collaboration with practi-
    tioners and educators,
    Sioux Valley Hospital,
    South Dakota, 127–28
Elderly. *See* Senior citizens
Energy
  consciousness as, 35
  disease as stalled or pene-
    trating, 21
  release of, for growth, 108
Engle, V. F., 51, 52
Entropy, 37n
  reversal of, 42, 46
Environment and person, in-
    teraction of as health, 17
Erwin, S. M., 63
Ethridge, P., xvii, 128

Evolution, 36–41
  of consciousness, 34, 36–41,
    43
  health as, 43–48
  disease as important to, 21
  pattern recognition as turn-
    ing point in, 41–43
  human, Young's theory of,
    xxvi, 42
Expanding consciousness, 33–
    48, 144, 145
  disease as, 23–24
  higher levels of, 66–68
  and HIV/AIDS phenomenon,
    22–23
  manifestations of, 51–68
  movement, 56–60
  time and timing, 53–56
Explicate order, Bohm's theory
    of, 10–11, 36, 62, 71

F

Family and community pat-
    terns of health and
    disease, 25–29, 115
Family nurse (FN), 132–33
Farnham, P. C., 63
Ferguson, M., 11–12
FN (Family nurse), 132–33
Freedom, Young's theory of,
    43, 44–46
Friedman, H. L., 63
Fromm, E., 137
Fryback, P. B., 23–24
Fuller, R. B., 21

G

Gaudiano, J., 51
Gendlin, E. T., 107

Gottlieb, R., 57
Grof, S., xvi
Guba, E. G., 87

H

Hall, R. L., 58, 59
Hart, L. A., 42
The Healing Web, 128, 131
Health
  as absence of disease, 3–4,
    134
  of community, 29
  as consciousness
    evolution of, 43–48
    expanding, formulation of
      concept of, xv, xxi–xxvi,
      51–52, 144
  continuum of, 4, 5
  disease as aspect of, 5–12,
    143
  family and community, pat-
    terns of, 24–29
  and illness, dichotomous
    view of, eliminating, 5–
    7
  paradigms of, 3–13
  as pattern of the whole, xix,
    10, 17–30, 82–83
  person-environment interac-
    tion as, 17, 44
  rhythmic fluctuations in, 11
  unitary process, 11, 82–85
  views of, 4–5
Health care, gap in, 122–24
Health care reform, xvii
  in New Zealand, 132–33
  and nurse as primary care
    provider, 139
  in United States, 133–34

Heart disease. *See* Coronary
    heart disease
Hegel, G. W. F., 6
Herman, R., 37n, 39–40
Hermann, N., 132
Heron, J., 85, 88, 116, 143–45
HIV/AIDS, 22, 23–24, 66
Hologram, 104–105, 107
Holographic model of inter-
    vention, 104–07
Holomovement, 10, 29, 83
Hospital
  bureaucratic system and
    time conflicts in, 53–56
  nurses' role in, 119–20, 145
Hypertension, 17
Hyperthyroidism, 17–19

I

Illness
  and health, dichotomy be-
    tween, eliminating, 5–7
  and patterns, reflected in,
    xxiii, 28
Implicate order, Bohm's theory
    of, xxvi, 10–11, 36, 56,
    74
Independent primary care pro-
    vider, 138–39
Information
  pain and disease as, 12
  of system, consciousness de-
    fined as, 33
Inquiry, cooperative, paradigm
    of, 85
Insider-expert, 114–15
Insight, 42
Instrumental paradigm, 12, 97

Integrating factor, disease as, 20–22
Interaction of consciousness via movement, 59–60
Intervention, 97–101, 102 (fig.)
  holographic model of, 104–07
  pattern recognition in, 86

J

Jantsch, E., 6, 34
Jarman, B., 140
Jones, R. S., 62
Jonsdottir, H., 20, 116

K

Keen, S., 106–07
Kinesthetic consciousness, 57
Kirlian photography, 19
Koerner, J., 127, 128
Kunz, Dora, 18, 19

L

Lamb, G. S., xvii, 55, 114, 116, 128, 129, 140
Lamendola, F., 20, 66, 103
Land, G., 21, 120, 140
Language, rhythm in, 58–59
Lather, P., 93
Leonard, G., 58
Lerner, L., 23
LeShan, L., 65
Light, whole from which universe evolved, 43
Lincoln, Y. S., 87
Litchfield, M., 109, 113, 114, 116, 132, 133
Love
  as consciousness, expanded, 67
  knowing as highest form of, 106–07
  unconditional, 104

M

Marchione, J. M., 99
Martin, M., 112
Matter
  as consciousness, manifestation of, 36
  determinate, 43–44
McDougall, W., 40
McWhinney, W., 22
Mechanic, D., 139
Medical paradigm, 107, 126
Meleis, A., 101
Mentzer, C., 51
Michaels, C., xvii, 55, 128, 129
Mikunas, H., 57
Mishel, M. H., 39, 101, 116
Moccia, P., 129
Moch, S. D., 20, 66, 85, 89
Moore, T., 140–41
Morgan, G., 93
Morphic resonance, 41
Morphogenetic fields, 40–41
Moss, R., xi, xxvi, 17, 19, 21, 23, 29, 30, 68, 97, 101, 141, 145
Moustakas, C., 87
Movement
  and consciousness, integration via, 56–60
  environment, control of, 46
  pattern of, 57–58
  rhythm and, 62
  and space-time, 46, 59–60, 63
Movement-time-space as mani-

Movement-time-space (*cont'd.*)
    festations of conscious-
    ness, 51–68
Muses, C., 33

N

NANDA (North American
    Nursing Diagnosis Asso-
    ciation), 86
NCM. *See* Nurse Case Manage-
    ment (NCM)
Nelson, J., 132
Newman, M., xv, xviii, 13, 20,
    51, 52, 55, 59, 61, 65, 66,
    81, 82, 99, 103, 122, 125,
    126, 129, 143–45
Nightingale, F., xvii
North American Nursing Diag-
    nosis Association
    (NANDA), 86
Nurse case management
    (NCM), 114–115, 145
  at Carondelet St. Mary's
    Health Center, 128–29
  and health care reform, 132–
    33
  partnership of clients, nurses
    and other health profes-
    sionals, 130–32, 145
Nurses becoming partners,
    130–32
Nurse-client relationship, 112–
    116, 129
  "being" with client, 103, 104
  caring, 140–42
  Carondelet St. Mary's Health
    Center, 128–29
  mutuality in, 84–85
  rhythm, 112–16
  timing, 129

Nursing
  cycles of change in, xvii–
    xviii, 120–22
  education. *See* Education
  home care, 55, 120
  hospital, 120–21
  integrative model of, 124–28,
    130
  intervention. *See* Interven-
    tion
  in paradigm, new, 107, 138–
    39
  primary, 121–22
  research. *See* Research
  team approach to, 121
Nursing role, 124–28
  clinician/case manager, 125,
    126, 145
  independent primary care
    provider, 138–39
  paradigms of, 125–26
  staff, 126
  team leader, 126
Nursing science, paradigm of,
    xviii, 81–93
  unitary-transformative per-
    spective, 20

O

Objective, concept of, 85
Objective time, 61
Oliveri, 29
Ostrander, S., 19

P

Paradigm shift, 12–13
Paradigms
  instrumental, 12, 97
  new, 138
  from old to new, 119–134

of interconnectedness, 113
medical, 107, 126
nursing, 107, 138–39
person-oriented, 126
of practice, 125–26
relational, 13
unitary-transformative. *See*
     Unitary-transformative
     paradigm
Parse, R. R., 82
Parsons, T., 4
Partnership with client, nurse
     entering into, 97–101
Patient care, temporal patterns
     in, 55–56
Pattern(s), xvi, 12, 52
  characteristics of, 72
  of consciousness, expanding,
     133
  crisis causing change in, 28–
     29
  disease as, 22–23
  evolution, role in, 41
  explicate manifestations of,
     71
  inquiry, methods of, 76–78,
     85
  methodology of, 71–78
  of movement, 57–59
     in families, 114, 115
  and quantity and quality,
     measures of, 72–73
  recognition of, 73–76
  temporal, in patient care, 55
Pattern of the whole, xix, 10,
     17–30, 24 (fig.), 73, 81–
     82, 86, 134
  individual-family-community
     as, 24, 25–29
Pattern recognition, xvii, xxvi,
     73–76, 85, 92, 107–09, 114

in evolution of conscious-
     ness, 41–43
nurse-client relationship, 129
research methodology, 85–
     88, 147–48
Patterning, characteristics of,
     72
Peck, M. S., 67
Pelletier, K. R., 20, 109–10
Person-environment
  evolving pattern of, 33
  interaction, disease as, 17, 44
Person-oriented health para-
     digm, 126
Physician's assistant, 138
Piaget, J., 59
Polkinghorne, D. E., 87–88
Presentational construing, 88
     90, 92
Prigogine, I., 37–40, 64, 102
     (fig.)
Primary nursing, 121–22
Primm, P. L., 127
Process wisdom, 77
Propositional construing, 88–
     89
Psychosis, 20

Q

Quinn, J. F., 113

R

Ravitz, L. J., 19
Real Nurses, 122
Reality, 35, 36, 61–62, 67
Reed, P. G., 47
Reiss, D., 29
Relational paradigm, 13, 97
Remen, R. N., 23

Research, 81–85
  as praxis, xviii, 92–93
Reynolds, C. L., 81
Rhythm, 84, 109–12
  biological, 11
  health, rhythmic fluctuations
    in, 11
  in language, 58–59
  and movement, 58, 59–60
  nurse-client relationship, 129
  in talking, 58–59, 110
Rogers, M. E., xviii, xxiv–xxv,
    7, 12, 21, 22, 36, 71, 81
Rusch, S. C., 128

S

Schlotfeldt, R. M., 122
Schmitt, N. A., 84–85
Schorr, J. A., 51, 52, 63
Schroeder, L., 19, 52
Schubert, P. E., 114
Seagel, S., 57
Self-concept, space-time as in-
    dicator of, 63–64
Senior citizens, 60, 66, 128
Sheldrake, R., 40–41
Silences, attending to, 110–11
Sime, M., xviii, 52, 82
Sioux Valley Hospital, South
    Dakota, 127
Smith, A., 61
Smith, C., 109
Smith, M. J., 85
Society, similarity of, to dis-
    sipative structures, 39–
    40
Space-time
  beyond, 60
  binding of, 64
  and movement, 63–64

restriction of movement and,
    59–60
  expansion of, 61–65
Space-time-movement as mani-
    festation of conscious-
    ness, 51–68
Stempel, J. E., 114, 116, 140
Stengers, I., 37
Stephens, G., 53
Stone, H., 21
Subjective, concept of, 85
Subjective time, 61
Suffering and movement to
    higher level of con-
    sciousness, 142

T

Talking, rhythm in, 58–59, 110
Team approach in nursing, 121
Teilhard de Chardin, Pierre,
    xxv
Temporal pattern in patient
    care, 55
Tension characteristic of dis-
    ease, 21–22
Tetra group, 131–32
Therapeutic touch, 113
Thomas, L., 4, 5
Thompson, W. I., 22
Tiller, W. A., 19
Time
  and causality, 62
  and consciousness, relation
    to, xvi, 51, 53–56
  and explicate order, 62
  freedom from, 47
  and nursing care, effective-
    ness of, 55–56
  objective, 61

perception, 62
subjective, 61
and timing, nurse-client rela-
    tionship, 129
Time-space-movement as mani-
    festation of conscious-
    ness, 51–68
Tommet, 26
Tompkins, E. S., 51, 59
Transcendence, 46, 47, 63, 65
Transformation, personal,
    xviii, 129
Turning point, 65–66

U

Ubell, E., 4
Unitary human beings, Roger's
    theory of, xviii, xix, xxv,
    7, 81–82
Unitary-transformative para-
    digm, 20, 82–85, 139,
    140
  education based on tenets
    of, 127–128
  method, 85–88
  nursing case managers at
    Carondelet St. Mary's
    Health Center, Arizona,
    129
  and post-positivist approach,
    52
  presentation of theory, 88–
    92
  research, 51–52

University of South Dakota,
    128

V

Vail, J., 86
Vaill, P. B., 76, 77
Vaughan, F. E., 104

W

Walker, L. O., 81–82
Watson, J., 4, 101, 110–12, 138
Watson, L., 21, 41
Weber, R., 18
Wellness, high-level, 4, 5
West, M. C., 68
Wheeler, C. E., 92
Whyte, L. L., 41
Whole seen in parts, paradox
    of, 75
Wholeness, 83
Wilber, K., xxiv, 43
Wisdom, process, 77

Y

Young, A. M., xxvi, 19, 99
  consciousness, theory of
    evolution of, 41–48
  spectrum stages
    Binding, 64, 90, 92
    Centering, 66, 90, 92
    Choice point, 92, 99, 129